All the F*cking Mistakes

All the F*cking Mistakes

A GUIDE TO SEX, LOVE, AND LIFE

GIGI ENGLE

ST. MARTIN'S
GRIFFIN

First published in the United States by St. Martin's Griffin, an imprint of St. Martin's Publishing Group

www.stmartins.com

Part of chapter three was originally published in an article titled "Why No One Cares About the Stupid Thing You Did While Drunk" in March of 2016 on www.elitedaily.com.

Part of chapter twelve was originally published in an article titled "I Was the Other Woman" on May 19, 2017 at www.marieclaire.com.

Part of chapter fourteen was originally published in an article titled "Why Being Single Helps You Find 'The One' Faster Than Serial Dating" on June 27, 2017 at www.ravishly.com.

Designed by Susan Walsh

Library of Congress Cataloging-in-Publication Data

Names: Engle, Gigi, author.
Title: All the f*cking mistakes: a guide to sex, love, and life / Gigi Engle.
Other titles: All the fucking mistakes
Description: First Edition. | New York: St. Martin's Griffin, 2020.
Identifiers: LCCN 2019037611 | ISBN 9781250189738 (paper over board) |
    ISBN 9781250262332 (ebook)
Subjects: LCSH: Women—Sexual behavior. | Sex instruction. | Conduct of life.
Classification: LCC HQ29 .E54 2020 | DDC 306.708—2dc23
LC record available at https://lccn.loc.gov/2019037611

Our books may be purchased in bulk for promotional, educational, or business use. Please contact your local bookseller or the Macmillan Corporate and Premium Sales Department at 1-800-221-7945, extension 5442, or by email at MacmillanSpecialMarkets@macmillan.com.

First Edition: January 2020

10 9 8 7 6 5 4 3 2 1

To my family, who has always supported and loved me,
even when I decided to write about blow jobs for a living.

And to my husband, who changed everything.

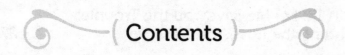

Contents

Part III: Let Me Save You the Trouble: Finding the Love You Deserve   277

INTRODUCTION
Let's Get Nasty

"Mommy?" A little girl looked up at her mother, eyes burning with deep, six-year-old contemplation. "Am I a nasty woman? Mommy, am I nasty? What does *nasty* mean?" She was probably five or six, had a head full of dark hair, and was wearing a purple dress with mismatched socks.

It was mid-election season. You know, before the world went to shit and a literal self-proclaimed sexual predator slithered into the White House like a slug.

The bb must have seen it on CNN, NBC, or (please, God, no) Fox News or something. Kids are chill as fuck these days. They watch the news. They know what's what. (A twelve-year-old I babysat once used the word *lit* and had his own Instagram.) The word *nasty* had, by mid-2016, unintentionally (or perhaps intentionally) infiltrated the mainstream. The kids wanted to know what the fuck was up. (Sidenote: Me, too, kiddo. Me, too.)

The little girl's mother knelt down to face her, brushing a stray piece of hair from her forehead. They both wore mismatched socks. The definition of #GOALS. I stopped scrolling through my own meme-tastic Instagram feed, suddenly anxious to hear the mother's response. *Lady, what are you going to tell this girl-child about Nasty? I gots to know. The f train is comin'.*

Her mother squeezed her hand and said, "It means we're doing things better than the men. It means we're getting stuff done."

The train arrived, and the two were whisked away in a sea of bodies. I'd later see this exact scene immortalized in an internet meme. Well, not the same mother and daughter—that would be fucking wild—but a very similar cartoon mother and daughter on one of those '50s-looking meme-ads. All good things become memes. I guess a lot of nasty women were explaining their nastiness to their young and impressionable children during the late summer of 2016. This all happened when there was still a lot of hope in the world. HRC was slaying, and women everywhere were starting to feel like the glass ceiling was inches away from being obliterated and the Patriarchy wasn't the ginormous clusterfuck we all know it to be.

As I stepped onto the train, service to social media lost (thanks, tunnel system), I had to ask myself, *What is a nasty woman? What is it really? Like, what are we even trying to convey here, y'all?* We can't fully identify what it means to be a nasty woman in the modern world without knowing what it means.

The definition of *nasty* is "highly unpleasant or nauseating." It means "gross, disgusting, or vile." You definitely don't want to put something nasty in your mouth (unless you do, which in that case, do your thing, fucker). Nasty means "bad." It means "straight-up shitty."

Isn't it delightful that the word would be used to describe a powerful woman running for the highest office in the land? How quaint, right? How charming.

Nasty has taken on a new meaning in our cultural lexicon. It is entirely feminized. It's a word used by men to describe women who aren't quietly abiding by the status quo. It's used to label any

woman who dares to open her fucking mouth and have an opinion. It describes those women who are owning their power, their
fierceness, and their sexuality. It's for women who give zero fucks
about what you think and all the fucks about their own fucking.
It's a negative word that is utilized by the Patriarchy to bring down
women who are making shit happen. And it won't work. Why?
Because we own that word. We may have "lost" the election, but
I hate to break it to you, White Twitter, we are still fucking here.

I'm sure as hell a nasty bitch. You tend to get grouped with the
nasty women when you write about blow jobs, vaginas/vulvas, and
orgasms for a living. When you're a woman with an eggplant emoji
as part of her Instagram bio, when you're a woman who speaks up
about sex, shit gets real.

What I do is considered tacky, gross, and tasteless. Society does
not like that I write about the taboo. Society is not a fan of sexual
openness. Society is fucking scared of a sexually open woman.
And society is not just out and about in the churches, steeples, and
streets. Society is online and in HD.

You know what I'm talking about here, Mama. Being a woman
on the internet puts you on the shitlist of every troll out in the ether.
You know the drill: You tweet your opinion about, I don't know,
doing laundry or the weather or your mom's new cat, Carl's Jr.,
and then some random dude with no avatar photo calls you a dirty
feminazi whore. We're constantly subjected to harassment, threats,
and emotional distress. The way the internet writes about women
in general is abhorrent. 4chan, Twitter, and Reddit subthreads have
transformed the World Wide Web into a garbage fire. Not that this
hasn't been happening forever. People have been spewing endless
streams of verbal diarrhea since the dawn of the internet. Shout-
out to AOL chat rooms (but also not, because that shit was hell).

The internet is a constant deluge of insults and vitriol; a hot, steaming shitpile of every self-indulgent piece of buttcrust who believes they were wrongly deprived of a chance to speak their minds. It's not a fun place. No one will help you. No one gives a fuck. You have to develop a thick skin to hack it. You have got to be nasty.

If you're nasty, this book is for you. If you're not nasty but are thinking, *Hey, maybe I could be, I don't know,* this book is also for you. You are a sexual woman, but you're even more than that. You're a complete, incredible, and whole human being. Your sexual empowerment does not define you; it just adds to your forceful spirit. You like to fuck, but you also like to work. You like to get some and get paid. You like to run your mouth and run fuckboys out of town. Only you can define yourself. You just need the tools to learn how to make that shit happen.

This book is a guide to taking your power back. It's for women who love sex and want that sex to be a source of strength. It's your antidote to the misogyny you've experienced for your entire life (some of which you probably aren't even aware of). It's the manual to understanding your worth and accepting that your sexual history has no bearing on your quality as a human. You are a shining beacon of strength. If you are comfortable with who you are and aren't afraid of that awesomeness, you can be whoever the fuck you want to be. No one can stop you, and no one can scare you into submission. You'll be able to advocate and fight for yourself in every facet of your life—whether it be your job, relationships, friendships, hookups, or a random interaction at the local corner store with some shitbag who tells you to "smile."

This book is for horny, badass sluts who want a raise, a raise right to the fucking top. Maybe with a dildo in hand. No judgment, Ma.

The lessons within these pages will teach you how to give yourself an orgasm *and* recover from an alcohol-induced shame spiral; how to tell a creepy douchebag to fuck off *and* how to fully explore fetishes like a dom-queen-slut-princess. You'll be able to explain the ins and outs of sex toys *and* cope with heartbreak if and when it comes. We're the future leaders of the world through our collective, insanely rad nastiness.

We have got to be like that phenomenal mother-daughter duo on the train. We've got to take back our lives and kick a bunch of ass so we can teach our daughters (and our sons) to do the same.

We've got this fire lit under our asses. We've got to make shit happen. If the last few years have taught us anything, it's that we've got to do this shit ourselves. Let's get nasty.

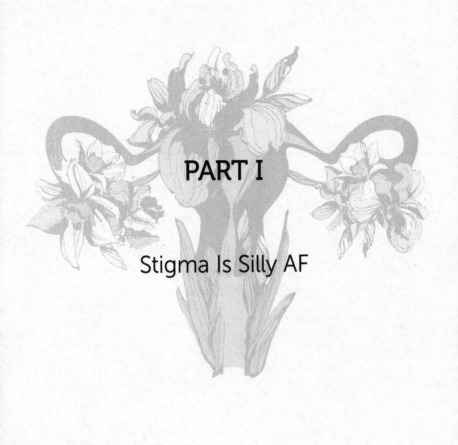

PART I

Stigma Is Silly AF

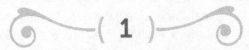

Sexual Empowerment in a World That Isn't Into It

I started having sex on the early side, according to standard cultural norms. At least, I felt like and feel like it was early to be fuckin'. You know, because sex (especially sex before marriage—thanks, most religions) is bad and we shouldn't do it. I was fifteen years old when I first had P-in-the-V intercourse. I had read more romantic novels growing up than I can count, so naturally I thought I understood just how love was supposed to be. My mother had raised me on Danielle Steel movies. I was the expert up in this bitch. Me and my low-cut, pink-and-black-striped (horizontal stripes, obvs) tank top and black hoop earrings were ready for this thing called love. Like many a horny sixth grader, I had my sexual awakening while reading Judy Blume's *Forever* and watching *Titanic*. Ugh, Leo. Be still, my loins.

So when I fell in love with my brother's heartthrob hunk of a best friend, lost my virginity on a beach, got a yeast infection (which I didn't tell him about), and then was dumped all within a six-month period during my freshman year of high school, it felt both cruelly surprising and startlingly on point. He even started dating one of my best friends shortly afterward. It was some classic

YA novel shit; it was a scene out of *All My Children*. I listened to a lot of Avril Lavigne that spring. All the Avril Lavigne, actually. (I'd originally written, "more Avril than I'm proud of," and then I realized I'm not ashamed of this at all. Long live Avril.)

In true teen-drama fashion, I had a lot of sex that summer with a lot of guys I didn't know very well, and, in some cases, not at all. There was a guy on a cruise ship to Alaska, standing up outside of a small library alcove. He came on the bottom of my dress, and it wasn't pleasant in any way. I walked around with come on my dress for, like, three hours, and no one seemed to notice. There was a guy in Switzerland who knew zero English except for the word *music,* and he had big blue eyes. There was a virgin from my ritzy north shore hometown who snuck into my house in the dead of night when everyone else was asleep, part of a great deflowering wherein I collected V-Cards like they were Berger's quest for the full deck in *Sex and the City*.

It was the summer that began my slut-dom. I was delightfully oblivious to all the negativity my actions were bringing down upon my reputation. When I say I was blissfully unaware of the anger and disapproval I was igniting in people around me, I say that earnestly. I was very aware of the sexual power I possessed, but not educated in the possible backlash. I used the sexual desire of boys for my own validation while I explored my power as a woman. I equated being wanted sexually with being worthy of love: a classic female blunder, born of patriarchal influence. I was a child with the same juvenile hubris of Molly Bloom in the opening scenes of *Molly's Game*. Read: an asshole. I could do no wrong. I was just living my life.

I was also heartbroken from my first boyfriend and was using sex as a way to cope with that pain. I figured I had already lost my virginity. It was to someone I loved, and so what difference could it possibly make to just keep fucking? I'd followed the rules, hadn't I? Hadn't I, Mom?!??!

Many girls have their first experiences with slut-shaming out of the blue. They haven't done anything remotely slutty (which is not to say that being slutty is bad; it is not). This was not the case for me. I had done all (most? All? I don't know?) of the things I was accused of, but that didn't make me any less angry. It didn't make the shaming any less fucked up.

What I missed was that people talked, they judged. People love to hate sluts. *Love* it. Teenagers (and their parents, I expect) loved to talk about me that summer. I was the hot gossip—me, my vagina, and my largely untouched clitoris. I guess I missed the memo that my sexual encounters wouldn't stay between myself and the boys I had fucked. I certainly didn't think my close girlfriends would sabotage me and tell my secrets. We may have been years away from learning about Shine Theory (which establishes that being around successful women benefits your own success), but come on.

I grew up in an old house across the street from West Park in a Chicago suburb. The park was where many of the local teenagers hung out; we were too young for bars and too old for the rec center, so we hung out in parks (or patches of surrounding trees and shrubbery). There wasn't anything else to do when school was out.

It was the beginning of summer. I was walking across the park when a boy I'd known during childhood (our moms had been friends) started screaming, *"Slut!"* at me from a bench. He didn't stand. He didn't chase me. He just sank his ass into the wooden bench and scream-shamed me. He kept screaming it at me across my journey over the field, until I reached my gate. I didn't register what had happened or even what had been yelled at me until I got inside. I didn't even flinch. I didn't respond.

This was a defining moment. It is the first time I remember being slut-shamed. It likely wasn't the first time, but it was the first time it clicked.

It was the moment I realized I wasn't powerful or infallible. All it took to bring down my unaware, inflated ego was an insecure boy screaming at me from across a stretch of grass. Looking back, I wish I had turned around and shouted back, "Listen, you little motherfucker, I am fresh off the boat of newly discovered sexual maturation, and I am trying to get my pussy wet in ways your bitch ass couldn't even fathom."

What I actually did was walk away in a pretty dignified manner, from what I remember. Obvs, I cried about it that night, but only my mom saw, so it doesn't count. Oh, wait, she fully called up that turd's mom and stood up for me, so it does count. It's okay, Mom. You meant well. Thanks for having my back.*

I still harbor a lot of resentment toward that kid. Every time my mom mentions some new failure he's had in his life (I hear there have been many. You know who you are, bitch!) or I glimpse a photo of his expanding waist and receding hairline, I feel a wave of satisfaction. My pettiness knows no limits, and I am happy I live in a world where the glorious art that is being petty has come home to roost. The point being, this moment stuck with me.

This is just one example that illustrates the darker side of how our culture perceives sexuality. Over a decade has passed, and it often feels like nothing has changed. Sex is still so shrouded in

---

* Sidenote: Moms are dope.

shame and stigma that we can't even talk about it, save for thinly veiled euphemisms, eggplant emojis, and/or painfully awkward exchanges.

Here we are as a society. We are almost totally and completely sex-negative, even when we do hail Samantha Jones for loving dick and Denise on *Master of None* for being the Master of Pussy. We're still fucked up about sex.

Beyond the overarching reality of sex negativity as a whole, we loathe the idea of sexual empowerment, especially in female sexuality. We hate the idea of a sexually free woman. A woman who slays peen or pussy is not chill. Don't even try to shake your head right now. Don't you even try to tell me I'm wrong. Yeah, Samantha Bee, Mindy Kaling, and Chelsea Handler are on television. Marginal, miniscule representation doesn't mean the world is suddenly into women being sexually free. I swear to God, I will scream, *"Burn the Patriarchy!"* at you for an hour if you shake your head. We elected a white man who brags about sexual assault as the president of the United States in 2016. Congress is jovially voting on whether or not we have the right to our own uteruses. My phone is blowing up with crisis alerts from Planned Parenthood because they are freaking out about their funding. Them's just the facts. Here we are.

WHY THIS BOOK NOW?

It's past goddamn time to topple the motherfucking Patriarchy. I'm not going to dance around it. This is post #MeToo and Time's Up. We've had e-fucking-nough. We're finished with this shit. It's time to be the badasses we are. Sexual empowerment is how we take back the power. It's how to fuck shit up.

Feminism has always been important, needed, and valuable, but in this particular current cultural diarrhea swirly, we have a dire need for a distinctly feminist understanding of sexuality. Sexuality must be equally valued and upheld, regardless of gender, for women to have equal rights. Sexuality must be accepted as a part of the human experience before we can have equal rights. Sex and feminism are bound.

Now, before you blow a hot angry load all over my chin, Jonathan, let's talk about the F-word.

FEMINIST ROOTS: WHY THE BAD REPUTATION?

Feminist has gotten a bad rep. It is a dirty word. When you hear the word *feminist*, it is almost always equated with "man-hating," "misandry," "white-man-blaming," "sexless female iconography," "self-imposed celibacy because men are fucking evil twats," and so on. You'd think we had MEN ARE GARBAGE tattooed to our foreheads.

Feminism is a poignant and important-as-fuck word, and to understand it (and why we need it), we have to take a look at its history. At the turn of the twentieth century, the word *feminism*— and the movement associated therein—was concerned primarily with legal issues: In the United States, the first wave was structured around giving women the right to vote and own property. You know, shit every fucking human should be able to do. The first wave hit its peak with the passage of the Nineteenth Amendment to the Constitution of the United States, which gave women the right to vote. First-wave feminist heroes include Margaret Sanger (who popularized the term *birth control*), Ida B. Wells (one of the founders of the NAACP), and Susan B. Anthony (most known for her work on women's suffrage).

Second-wave feminism arrived in the '60s, building on this foundation and adding to the ticket domestic violence, marital rape, and reproductive rights. Betty Friedan wrote *The Feminine Mystique* (1963), the book known for sparking second-wave feminism. In it, Friedan challenged the idea that women are happiest and completely fulfilled as housewives and mothers. And in 1968, the National Organization for Women (founded in 1966) successfully lobbied to pass a workplace-harassment amendment to the Civil Rights Act, which had been passed four years earlier. Second-wave feminist activists also worked with law enforcement to provide greater punishment for abusers.

Second-wave feminism was brought to an end over what is kind of the most hilarious thing ever: porn. One group split off, condemning porn as evil and degrading to women; the other was more narrowly pro-porn. The pro-porn feminists certainly saw the problematic nature of porn (a.k.a. the scripted coercion of women into sex acts, the strictly male lens, etc.)* but they recognized that it was entertainment, something that could be enjoyed by people of all sexes.

The pro-porn feminists won the war on porn. Let's face this shit—no one was ever giving up wanking to threesomes and anal.

---

* I once watched a clip with an ex-boyfriend where a guy tells a girl they're going to have anal, and she legit says, "No. I'm scared." And he responds, "It's something new. You'll love it," before sticking it up her bum. This was part of a script!

And why should they? Hey, I love a good anime gang bang on a casual Thursday night, you guys. One time, I rubbed one out to a sexy cartoon, girl-on-girl sex scene while my friends were getting ready to pregame for the bars in the next room. I hear that shit. Porn is a great form of entertainment. It was never going to be outlawed. Get real.

After everyone was like, "Okay, porn is great, and we're gonna keep rubbing our dicks and clits to it," third-wave feminism slid in with the same gusto with which a Wall Street guy adopts a coke habit. We love porn, guys. It's fine.

In the 1990s, the term *intersectionality* appeared, and the third wave washed in. Feminists called for the rights of *all* women—women of different nationalities, ethnicities, religions, and cultural backgrounds, who had often previously been ignored by or straight-up excluded from white feminism.

The feminist shit-talkers of the right-wing, conservative, values-driven, ass-clown brigade are over here likening the whole of the modern feminist movement to the more extreme, "radical" second-wave feminist views of Germaine Greer and Mary King that coiled into the 1980s. Much of this backsliding is because those in opposition to feminism think we believe men are all human trash. This is the "matriarchy" bullshit rhetoric that lingers on the tongues of those opposing a feminist outlook today. They are terrified we're going to come in and create an underground slave world where the men are forced to live and are only brought into the sunlight when we need their jizz. I mean, God forbid a movement evolves and changes over time, right?

Additionally, the idea that we want rights for *all women* is scary as fuck because the idea of women having equal rights feels like fewer rights for the men. That is what fucking privilege does to people—someone gaining the same rights you have feels personally oppressive.

THE POWER STRUGGLE AND WHY IT MAKES SO MANY DICKS SOFT

Here is something you need to get about feminism, something you need to drill into your mind: We don't want to take power away from men so we can have it and collect it into our shrew-caves along with all the many stolen children and cats. It blows my fucking mind that we are still fighting for equal treatment in all aspects of life, but, as I said, here we are.

Let me be crystal clear here. We *do* want to take some specific power away from men. We do. We fucking do.

The only time we want power taken away from men is when it is holding us down. We want it stripped away when it gives male coworkers more money for the same work, allows them to undress us with their eyes, pressure us into sex we have but don't want, and gives social permission to tell us we look sexy in those shorts. A man should not be able to touch a female coworker's thigh and face zero repercussions. You shouldn't be able to comment on someone's body on the street without getting called out for your bullshit. Asking for shitty, aggressive, threatening behavior to be checked is not too much to ask for. If you think it is, you can fuck off. When men complain about feminism, it's like, "It's outrageous that we can't treat women like shit anymore! We can't grab a single ass! We can't grope as we wish! We can't comment on anyone's low-cut top! It's PC culture gone mad, I tell you!" It feels like the women are threatening an underground slave market for the men because that's what the Patriarchy wishes it could do to women.*

FEMINISM IS EQUALITY. ARE YOU INTO IT OR WHAT?

Feminism, by definition, is equality between the sexes. Feminist sexuality means sexuality that is equal. Feminist sexuality means forging a view of sexuality that doesn't differentiate male versus female. We need to look at sex as a whole, rather than as two different entities, judged by two different sets of standards. Had a teenage boy been slaying as hard as I had in the summer of '09, he would have been a stud. All the girls would have wanted to date him, and all the boys would have wanted to be him. I was labeled a slut. My stock was shot. You don't have to be a rocket scientist to see how fucked up it is that we think like that. Sexual inequality is rampant in the very foundation of our thinking as humans. We need to change the way we think about women and sex.

We need to reassess how we categorize female sexuality. That is the mission.

The truth is, women like to fuck. Women like to come. We just need the rest of the world to fucking get that shit. If you're looking for that potion to juice you up, the one that gives you the amped-up energy you need to be a badass woman in control of her sexuality; if you want to fuck who you want to fuck . . . you're in the right place.

---

* Secretly loving how many men are probably reading this and screaming, *"Feminazi cunt!"* into the void right now.

In case you've been living under a rock for the last, I don't know, forever, shit has gotten very real and not in a fun *Jersey Shore* reality TV kind of way. The gains we thought we'd made and solidified now seem more and more fragile. Progression for naught, we are still very much living in a world where a woman's body is politicized and up for regulation. It's like we've come full circle (jerk). Our reproductive rights are being voted on. *Roe v. Wade* is back on the table for discussion. We live in a world where two out of every three rapes go unreported.

(If you want to know why rape goes unreported, just look at the Bill Cosby trial. Sixty women come forward to accuse a man of sexual assault, and the jury can't decide if he actually assaulted anyone. I mean, he was finally brought to justice only after dozens of women accused, news stories exploded, and a retrial was demanded. Go figure. There are countless more cases just like this one. *cough* Brock Turner *cough*)

Ladies, nasties, fellow vagina owners. It has never been more important than right now to be a sexually empowered woman. Now is the time. We need to reclaim and own our sexual identities.

We need to say, "Fuck. That."

We take down the Patriarchy by taking back our sexual freedom. Or, I guess, taking it in the first place. Owning that motherfucking shit. Be a slut, don't be a slut, but do whatever the fuck you want.

Our bodies are regulated, given value, and consumed by men. We aren't given agency. If you break it down to these simple facts and lay the bones bare, there it all is. It's all about sex. It's all linked back to that day in the park when that boy called me a *slut* and made me cry.

When we take back sex, the patriarchal power we bow down to cannot make us bend. The threat is gone, the ammo is obliterated.

You can't control women when you take the chains off. When calling someone a *slut* has no effect, when not even feeling the need to make your partner come during sex stops being socially acceptable, one sex doesn't have the upper hand anymore.

Removing the chains, that is where it gets tricky, isn't it? Moving away from a lifetime of ingrained messaging and whore-shaming is not like getting a makeover at your local salon or going to school for a Ph.D. The path is not clear, especially when those in power are in no way going to hand some of it over willingly.

Yet breaking free and owning your power, your pussy power, is so significant and consequential to female liberation. Cidney G. Green, creator of the infamous viral internet video "Pussy Over Pain," once spoke on a panel called "The Policy of Pleasure versus Pain" at the Museum of Sex in New York City. The question asked was posed by panel moderator and *Teen Vogue* wellness editor Vera Papisova. It was something like: *How do we approach and talk to people who don't want women to have access to products that help them fully realize their sexuality and enjoy their bodies?*

Cidney, a powerful speaker, a striking black woman in short shorts and combat boots, took the mic. She said that if she were speaking to a man who said that women shouldn't have access to these products or access to her sexuality, she would have to say that she *chooses* to enjoy her sexuality and how it makes him *feel* is not her problem. She would say that whatever he was *feeling* about the way she engages in pleasure is not her issue. If it makes him uncomfortable, that is his problem, not hers. It is not our responsibility as women to change ourselves to fit the fancy of another person. How you choose to feel is your own business and is the only thing within your control. It is not our responsibility to make any other person feel good about themselves and feel happy in their own skin. We can only control how we feel and what makes us happy in *our* own skin.

That's where this entire guide comes in, to lead you (just a little), to hold your hand. It is the tool book you'll take with you on your journey of sexual discovery and exploration. It is chock-full of the sexy-ass lessons you'll utilize while burning the motherfucking Patriarchy to the ground. You know how we'll know when the male-centric bullshit is over? When any woman anywhere can fuck or not fuck whoever she wants without giving it a second thought, when rape culture ends, when women are free to be who the fuck they are without fear. That's the power of sexual freedom.

This is what we have to understand as women, as sexual creatures. This is where we have to begin. We are in control of our own feelings, of our own bodies, and our own happiness. Once we realize the raw power of this unrealized fact, we can move toward owning it, together, as women.

Bitch, you are killing *it*. Never for a second doubt your importance or your impact. You are the shit. Our sexuality is so potent and powerful. Our orgasms are legitimately endless. We don't have the same refractory periods as male-bodied people. You can come and come and come and never stop. We are a well of energy that is waiting to be unleashed. Think about how amazing the female body actually is. We're talking about a vessel that has the ability to grow a human inside of it and give life. We're talking about a vagina that can stretch to accommodate an infant's head and then return to form. The female body can slough away the endometrium, the lining of the uterus, bleeding for five days without dying. This is just what a woman can do without even trying. These are nature's simple add-ons. That is how powerful the female body is.

When she's using her brain, she can rule the whole damn planet. She can be anything and do anything she wants.

No wonder people are so terrified of women. No wonder we aren't told this shit. If we knew, we'd fuck everything up. Women are the most powerful creatures on the planet. We're fucking scary, and we're fucking magic.

When you have control over your sexuality, you are unstoppable. Now, before we get into this more extensively, we should look at the *why* more closely.

WHY FEMALE SEXUALITY IS SO FUCKING SCARY (AND WHY THAT'S BULLSHIT)

Unless you're on one of the coasts (and even then, a lot of the time), sex is considered bad, dirty, and impure—when it's actually natural, healthy, and amazing.

Women are told they are whores if they like sex, for the way they dress, and for saying no to unwanted sexual advances. Should a woman choose to abstain from sex, she's a moralist killjoy; she's no fun. It's like Allison says in *The Breakfast Club*: "Well, if you say you haven't [had sex], you're a prude. If you say you have, you're a slut. It's a trap. You want to, but you can't, and when you do, you wish you didn't, right?"

What a precarious position we ladies find ourselves in. There is actually no winning. You cannot win as a woman when you have these stringent, impossible standards in place. The Patriarchy has crafted a system.

So, I say again, fuck that.

A sexually free woman is the scariest thing in the entire world.

It is fucking mind-boggling. It is the screw that, when loosened and removed, topples the entire structure. How? Because we are controlled by sex. Every single inequity in this modern culture is based in sexist denial or straight-up demonization of female sexuality. We have to maintain our reputations and worry about our reputations constantly. We aren't free. The word *slut* is used to box us in. If you're a slut, you have no value. You're used and dirty. It's a slippery slope from hell. You should wear the low-cut top to score the man, but also a chastity belt because he's not going to marry you if you "give it up." When I was being called a slut and a whore in that park, I could feel my status declining. Even as a young kid, I knew my value was whether or not someone wanted to be my boyfriend. Look at Bailey Davis, the Saints' cheerleader who was fired for posting a sexy Instagram photo in 2018. She was the captain of the team until one misstep ruined her career. She didn't control her image as a sexy, untouchable woman. She was labeled an easy whore, so she became a worthless piece of rubbish that could be tossed into the fucking wind.

According to RAINN (the Rape, Abuse & Incest National Network), over 50 percent of college-aged women are sexually active. Yet the world demonstrates through sexual exploitation, rape culture, slut-shaming, and an emphasis on female "purity" that the world is *not* into women fucking. It's a multipronged approach: We're slut-shamed, we're whore-shamed, we're told to "cover up," and yet we're told we need to be physically beautiful to be wanted or valuable. Just like Bailey Davis, we're told to be sexy, but not slutty. Sexually attractive, but not sexually available. A 2011 study found that slut-shaming is a major problem in high school and even middle school, and it constitutes most sexual harassment cases in these places. In *Full Frontal Feminism*, author Jessica Valenti cites the "shut up, you ugly bitch" argument as a means of control: Young women are constantly reminded they're there to be ogled, and everything we have is based in how we look.

We're imbued with the message that it's our fault if we get raped because we shouldn't have been dressed like skanks. We're as worthy as our physical attractiveness, but also responsible for being attacked. As Valenti puts it, don't have sex, but be sexy. (And a million other things that make us feel shitty.)

We're told we're not "marriage material" if we have bad reputations. There is still a belief that a woman who has sex before marriage is not worthy of a husband. In some societies, women are still expected to bleed on their wedding night; if they don't, their new husbands believe they've been "betrayed." While this is an extreme example, we are locked into systems of sexual control by way of shame and servitude. Society would not like us to have total agency and control over our bodies.

Why? Let's be real, if we have control over our sexuality, we have control over our lives. Without slut-shaming, hymen obsession, promise rings, and purity balls, we break down some of the patriarchal power that bounds us. We are controlled by who we fuck or who we don't fuck.

If we allow other people to tell us what we're worth, we lose the ability to find our own worth and our own identity. It's like what Jill Filipovic writes in her essay "Offensive Feminism: The Conservative Gender Norms that Perpetuate Rape Culture, and How Feminists Can Fight Back": "When you extend human rights to women, they act like human beings with individual needs, ambitions, and desires—just like men."

If you take back sexuality and accept that every single human person is a sexual being, you create equality. If men and women are held to the same standards of sexual integrity, safety, and care for a partner, we can move into a new world. It sounds trite, but it's really that simple. Will sexual liberation end war and poverty? Probably not. But it will make the world a better place to live in for all people, everywhere.

PERSIST, PERSIST, PERSIST!

I spoke with many highly regarded, kick-ass women while I was researching this book. One of them is Dr. Tammy Nelson, a prominent sex therapist and author of many books, including *The New Monogamy*. She gave me some insight into what it means to take back our sexuality and why society frames sexuality so differently for boys and girls.

Dr. Nelson says that in today's world, we can't just say women have to *resist* everything that is happening to them right now. We have to *persist*. We have to step up and keep going. We can't stop fighting, only the fighting is not burning bras or starting the revolution with machine guns and other violent shit. The only blood we shed is period blood. And maybe in blood play.* It's in sexual autonomy. Finding joy in your sexuality and pleasure is its own form of persistence. It is resistance against the ideas that hold us back from realizing our true potential. Women have evolved and should continue to evolve toward a place where we know we deserve pleasure and demand it. We need to rule the world.

She is so right on. We do have to persist. We have to embrace our sexuality as a means of joy, confidence, happiness, and self-

---

* *Blood play* is a sexual fetish. We'll get to kink and fetish later.

worth. We have so much power that we don't even know exists within us; we must figure out how to utilize that power. Not to get woo-woo here, but we are the center of humanity and the vessels of human life. That is some formidable shit. Pussy power is no joke.

WOMEN ARE PROGRAMMED TO BELIEVE THEY AREN'T WORTH SHIT

We see more violence, murder, and death on television and in movies than we ever do sex. Just a few years ago, a study cited in *The Independent* found that seventy-four countries have bans on same-sex sexual contact. If we see a dick on television, we are goddamn scandalized. We cannot stop talking about it from Facebook to Twitter to Perez Hilton. *Did you see that giant uncircumcised penis on* Game of Thrones *last night?*

We don't think twice about violence. We are numb to guns, blood, and gore. We're fine with kids playing violent video games where they blow each other's heads off and bathe in zombie blood, but Lord help us if they see a clitoris or a ball sack. God forbid they see two people loving each other in a way that is inherently natural across the entire animal kingdom.

That is how we're taught to think about sex, as something worse than violence. It is dirtier than violence.

We're not concerned with violence when sex is the thing to control and codify. Girls are given fucked-up messages about sexuality from the time we're in diapers. *Rapunzel* teaches young girls that the only way to escape a kidnapping is with the help of a strong man. *The Little Mermaid* says that finding a man means losing your voice and giving up your family—and that this is a worthwhile trade to make. Fashion magazines tell young girls that if they aren't a size 2, with flawless skin and perfect hair, men won't want them. And if men don't want you, you are worthless.

This goes beyond sex-shaming. We take agency away from women in countless ways. Young women are brought up with the understanding that their bodies don't belong to them. Think about this shit for a second because we do it all the time. We tell children to "hug Uncle Tommy!" whether or not they want to hug Uncle Tommy. Never mind that Uncle Tommy is fucking creepy as shit. Mothers put daughters in princess costumes and buy them dolls, even though they might prefer to be a fucking cowgirl. They don't ask. We tell little girls that if a boy bullies them, it means they like them. We affirm abusive behavior instead of saying, "You should tell Billy to keep his fucking hands to himself. No one gets to touch you without asking." We don't give them the option of consent. We don't drive a sense of self-worth and self-ownership into young women.

While scrolling through my feed, avoiding deadlines, per usual, I saw a photo on a feminist author's Instagram; a repost from a father of himself, his daughter, and her prom date. The father was holding a gun. The caption read, "I hope my beautiful daughter and her date have a great time at prom." While this may be seen as a joke and a warning to her date to be a "gentleman," what it actually is is a reminder that this man perceives his daughter as his property. She can't protect herself. It is between himself and her date to decide her fate. She doesn't get a say. The date is the one who wants sex. She is not a sexual being.

Krystyna Hutchinson and Corinne Fisher cite a letter they received from a reader in their book, *F*cked,* wherein a young woman wasn't allowed to leave her house in shorts because her parents told her she might get raped. If she wore shorts, she'd be putting herself in danger. It would be her responsibility.

These are just a few examples. We have to acknowledge the kind of messages we're sending from all areas of life because that shit is fucking us in the ass with a black spiked dildo. And not in a good way. I'm talking lubeless ass-fucking.

Messages are given to us in a mixed-up, confusing way, from many different avenues—bombarding our senses, making it difficult to register the subliminal effects in all its fucked-up glory. It sounds very *X-Files*, but it's true. We see Nicki Minaj shaking her incredible ass, and we want to emulate that sexiness. We see Lady Gaga riding naked on a horse, and we want to be like her. At the same time, both of them are simultaneously shamed for being sluts, regardless of (or perhaps because of) their mega-talent and empowering messages to young women to own their bodies.* What we see is a clusterfuck, a mishmash of imagery and rhetoric that glamorizes sexiness and demonizes actual sex all at once.

I was given mixed messages as a kid when it came to sex. My mom wanted me to be sexually liberated but not to be a slut. There is a difference, mind you. As a little girl, I was told masturbation and nudity were normal and healthy. I understood that sexual feelings were something I inherently possessed, and I didn't fear those feelings.

At the same time, she also told me, "No one buys the cow if the milk is free." A leftover lesson from her strict Catholic upbringing by a militant librarian mother. I was taught that sex is a commodity, and it does not have a bottomless supply. If you give it away, you have less to give someone else. The more you give, the less you

---

* Not to mention Nicki always tells kids to stay in school. Which is a pretty fucking wholesome message.

have; the more used you are. This lowers your stock price. If your stock price is lower, you're less attractive to a potential suitor and therefore less likely to be valued at a price to become a prized wife and mother. If it sounds a lot like trading livestock at the county fair, à la *Charlotte's Web,* that's because it is basically the same thing.

The World Wide Web is another layer in this confusing shitshow. Sex sells, but advertisers won't go near sexually explicit content, which makes writing about sex harder to monetize, which makes paying qualified people to write about it harder to justify. When your company makes all its money off ads, but none of the sex content can have ads, it makes covering sex (that is, factual depictions of sex and pleasure) less appealing. When I worked at Thrillist Media Group (now Group Nine), I was led to believe I'd have boundless freedom to write about sex in a scientific, thorough, unencumbered way. I wanted to create worthwhile content that legitimized sexuality as a normal part of the human experience. If we could write about food, reality television, travel, and sports, we could write about sex.

For a time, I did have that loose leash. When the company made the big merger, the white men in charge decided they were too upscale to talk about something as dirty as sex. I was relegated to dating-only content until they eventually decided to cut the section from the site altogether. This is just an example of how the game can go. It's 2020, and we still fear sex so thoroughly that we avoid it in the name of decency, while simultaneously projecting hypersexualized images of half-naked females on every corner of the screen. Confusing, yes? Do we love sex? Do we hate it? I don't know!

Seriously, what the fuck are we supposed to do, guys?

These messages are further reinforced by emotionalized female sexuality—the "Waiting for Your Prince" motif, laid out by

Peggy Orenstein in her book *Girls & Sex*. Sex is the ultimate gift. It is something you give away to a man when you're in love. You give up your magical flower to a man (it is always a man in these heteronormative scenarios) who is worthy. Sex is not something you want because you're a horny teenager with flushed emotions coursing through your body.

No, that isn't how it works. Sex and love are two indefinable entities that are forever linked. If you don't wait for your prince to have sex, your prize is less worthy. If you don't have sex as a by-product of love, you aren't doing it correctly. You are cheapening yourself. You may never even find your prince because you are a big old whore now.

SEX AND EMOTION, THE FEMALE CLUSTERFUCK

When I asked Dr. Nelson about what it takes to be sexually liberated, she said that women need to not give their power up to their partner. When women cede sexual decisions to their partners, they lose agency—for example, when we compromise on having an orgasm (or downright fake it). We have to assume control of the power we have by realizing it's there. It isn't power to hand over; it's power to revel in.

We give up our power by not understanding our own erotic feelings. We give away our emotional power too quickly when we buy into the bullshit idea that our partner is what gives us value and by confusing sexual feelings for love.

When a girl feels attraction, she usually emotionalizes her sexuality automatically. Girls have been told that they don't just have sex for the sake of pleasure, because that makes them slutty. So, we think we love someone when what we really have is a hard-on for them. We legitimately confuse feelings of sexual desire with feelings of emotional love because we've been socially conditioned to think that we cannot have one without the other. It's a way to justify horniness. If we're told we can't have sex until we're in love or married, we subconsciously fabricate feelings of emotional love to make it okay in our own heads.

I thought I loved my first boyfriend. I wanted to have that romantic, movie-scene sexual experience with someone I loved. He was perfect. He looked like a fairy-tale prince and humped like a robot on crack cocaine. He screwed me dry on a mattress in a friend's bedroom in the middle of the afternoon. Those were the rules I was supposed to follow. I wonder how my sexual maturation might have been different if I had been taught to critically discern the difference between my clit tingling and feelings of love.

To be fair, first love isn't always born of horniness, but I'll take a bet that many times it is. When I was a rebellious, kind of douchey teenager, my mom would say that I didn't know what love was. She was damn right. I didn't know what love was, and I didn't know what horniness was. No one ever tells us these things. They never tell us the two can be intertwined or totally separate.

Here is the big problem in all this: If we tell girls that they have to wait around for someone to decide to be in a relationship with them so that they can fuck, it gives another person all the power. The yes must come from the other person. If the other person doesn't "lock it down," you have nothing.

SELF-AWARENESS IS THE KEY
TO SAYING, *"FUCK ALL!"*

In order to maintain control over our bodies, our desires, and our feelings, we have to be self-aware. It's about having the right information, the real information. I'm talking about understanding your clitoris, determining what you want out of a relationship, and knowing that your worth is entirely self-determined. Sexual autonomy is our ultimate source of power. Confidence, both sexually and on a more basic, human level, is what makes women powerful. These lessons start young. They need to begin right away.

In order to breed that power and confidence into women (and men), we have to provide accurate and comprehensive sex education. We have to teach children that sex does feel good, that it's okay to experience pleasure, and how to have it safely (if they decide they are emotionally ready for it).

We need to explain to girls how their bodies work. We have to encourage them to get to know their bodies. We need to show them diagrams of the clitoris and talk about the shit no one seems to want to explain. We can't pretend it isn't real.

Of course, that doesn't work. Something doesn't go away just because you lock it up and hide it. We are just a big ol' confused bunch of peeps who don't know what a clitoris is or how to not get our hearts broken by morons.*

Dr. Nelson reiterates that the only way to alleviate the colossal confusion around sex, the damaging messages kids are fed through

---

* Morons who high-key also don't know what a clitoris is, by the way.

the media, and the unfair emotionalization of sexuality is educating kids about sex and about desire.

You cannot understand your sexuality if you don't know how to engage with your sexuality. Whether we like it or not, desire runs the planet. It doesn't matter if you choose to suppress it or set it free, it still runs the planet. It is everything. It is in the very foundation of our beings. Regardless of gender, we have feelings of erotic desire within us. The feelings and emotions need to be integrated into what we learn about ourselves. Sexual desire and love are not one and the same. They can go together, but they don't have to all the time. You can have sex without feelings that can lead to feelings, or you can have feelings that then lead to sex.

Currently, we get little to no education about sex at all, let alone a curriculum that would allow us to garner the difference between erotic desire and love. We are so far from learning emotional intelligence it is laughable.

We need to educate about pleasure, consent, and STIs. Forgoing information does not stop people from fucking. It just stops them from doing it safely. I still get full-body chills when I think about my 106-year-old sex-ed teacher, in full muumuu regalia, putting a condom on a banana. That moment encapsulates my entire memory of sex ed. It was all heteronormative mechanics, all fearmongering, and no real useful information.

We're scared of teaching kids about the realities of sex because we're terrified of breaking up this system. We like our systems. They comfort us. Meanwhile, only thirteen states mandate that the sexual education taught in schools be factually correct. This means most U.S. schools have the option to teach information that is either only partially correct, omits information, or isn't based in science whatsoever. That is how much we fear sexuality.

An article from the April 2008 *Journal of Adolescent Health* found that teens with comprehensive sex ed are 60 percent less likely to wind up with an unplanned pregnancy, yet many states are teaching abstinence-only messages.

Want to know how many U.S. states require that educators mention anything about sexual pleasure when teaching about sex? None. Zero states require that we teach about pleasure. No one even has to say, "Sex feels good." No one seems to feel the need to say sex feels good. If they did, they could probably be fired.

I made this fact up, *but* I'd wager my right tit* that 99 percent of the times people engage in sexual activity, it is not for procreative purposes. We bang because it feels good. We just ignore this fact and pretend it isn't there because of that ingrained societal discomfort around sex. No one knows what a fucking clitoris is without either Googling it or discovering their older brother's electric toothbrush. We absolutely need to teach comprehensive, pleasure-based sexual education in school. Reproduction and reproductive safety are, of course, important and necessary, but making babies is not the only thing sex is about. We are doing girls and young people everywhere a great disservice by neglecting to teach them about their natural human urges.

Currently, there are girls who walk out of school having absolutely no idea how their bodies work, where their clitoris is, or what feels good. We're like: *Well, I guess sex is just a thing we have to do to make our partners happy. Le sigh.* What a life. Two in three women require clitoral stimulation (and probably more, according to recent research) to achieve orgasm, yet the clitoris is rarely (if ever) mentioned during sex education. A 2005 study found that 29 percent

---

* The right tit is the good one, too.

of college-aged students could not locate the clitoris on a diagram. Their failure to do so points directly back to a mismanaged sex-ed program in high school. All this is misinformation and omission is entrenched in those antiquated ideas about sexuality, promiscuity, and female pleasure.

ONE CLIT TO SAVE US ALL

In 2017, I did extensive research on the clitoris. I spoke to experts, read journals and studies, and finally wrote a piece for *Glamour* magazine covering the internal clitoris. Haven't heard of it? That's okay. Barely anyone has.

The medical community didn't figure out the clitoris goes far below the external, nubbin-like glans that you can see out on the outside of the vulva until—surprise, surprise—a female urologist named Helen O'Connell, M.D., figured it out while dissecting cadavers. She published her work *Anatomy of the Clitoris* in 1998. We didn't know about the full structure of the clitoris until two years before I wore a fully silver outfit to ring in the new millennium.

The clitoris is the female pleasure organ, not the vagina. *Vagina* is also the most misused word in the English language, probably. Don't google it. The powerhouse of female pleasure is the clitoris. The clit is homologous to the erectile tissue from which the penis is formed, contains eight thousand nerve endings, and it needs stimulation to produce female orgasm. Many studies have reported that fewer than 30 percent of women orgasm from penetration alone. This has a lot to do with how close the vaginal opening and the clitoris are. According to Dr. Wednesday Martin, an anthropologist and author of *Untrue*, if your clitoris is less than two inches from

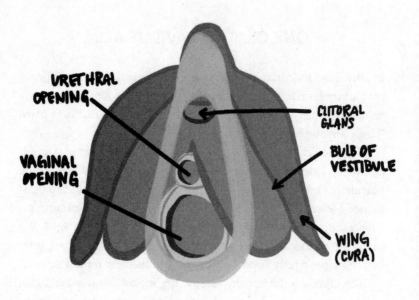

the vaginal opening, you're more likely to come during sex. The problem is that this is SUPER rare. To make matters even more confusing, studies that show that 30 percent of women can have orgasms during sex leave out positions like Coital Alignment Technique, wherein the clitoris is rubbed against the pubic bone, as well as the women who, within this study, were manually stimulating themselves or using a toy. During penetration, the clitoris is rarely reached. Even when it is and you have a vag-gasm, the clitoris is, at the very least, being indirectly stimulated through the anterior wall of the clitoris.* It sits quite a ways above the vaginal opening. If you don't know where a clit is, or how to touch it, you're not going to come.

This is the first step in releasing females from the stringent cadre of sexual servitude. Knowing your anatomy and how to properly label it helps you take back your power and own your sexual pleasure. If you can rely on no one but yourself to make yourself come, you're on par with the men.

Men run the world, so we cater to them. Boys are taught that their pleasure is a given. Hetero sex is over when a dude comes. Orenstein cites several interviews in *Girls & Sex* with teenage girls, noting the frequency with which these girls readily handed out blow jobs. Most of the girls reported that a blow job was "no big deal," but they never expected oral sex in return. They cited it as something for "long-term" relationships.

This Blow Job Paradox is a poignant example of how we view female sexuality.

We're never taught about female desire. Girls are never taught that they can experience pleasure in the same way a boy can.

---

* More on that later.

Remember the livestock analogy wherein sex is the commodity for sale? This is why no one teaches you about the clitoris or about female pleasure. If you figured out you were a human being and that sex and your pussy were things that actually *do* replenish themselves infinitely, how the hell could anyone control you? We must maintain the illusion.

When you take all this bullshit into account, and look at the big, fucked-up picture, it is frustrating, but it isn't your fault. It's what you've been conditioned to believe about sex. The only place to turn is the computer. If no one is going to tell you anything, media seems like the best option.

GIRLS AND PORN AND PORN AND GIRLS

The internet is where we all have to find out about our bodies. It's the only place we have to go. If parents aren't having conversations about sex and pleasure, and neither are teachers, kids are out of options.

The internet has the potential to give you endless resources, as long as the media decides to cover sex in a responsible and scientifically accurate manner. At the same time, it is also one massive porn search engine.

When I was about eight, I searched the word *vagina* on whatever rudimentary search engine my family's colorful-ass Mac computer (remember those?) had at the time. Internet Explorer, maybe? Whatever. What was more offensive than the slow-as-shit dial-up internet connection was the images it produced: tiny blond women everywhere with their pussies being smashed by giant monster cocks. I was traumatized as fuck by that. I had never seen sex before. I didn't even know what it was, and here I was at far too young an age, witnessing double penetration and anal sex from penises the size of horse dongs. I should not have been seeing that as a small child. That's fucked up.

Porn is entertainment. It is highly stimulating and can be highly arousing. That doesn't make it an accurate depiction of real-life sex. We have to relay this to young people so that they understand that. Without proper sex education, they wind up with porn. And porn, though entertaining and somewhat inspiring, glamorizes bodies to the point of obscuring real qualities, like pubic hair or cellulite: the things that make us human and therefore vulnerable. Porn becomes the only thing young people have. And if all you know is porn, you're going to be surprised and maybe a little disappointed by your first real sexual encounter—not to mention altogether bad at sex. Porn stars don't pay attention to the clitoris. They pop from anal to vaginal sex on a whim. This is both unrealistic and dangerous.

Do you want your kid to think that sticking a penis into an asshole, sans lube, and then straight into a vagina, while another dude is also getting a blow job is the way people have sex? Learning sex through porn is like learning how to be a good employee by watching *Office Space*. It's the same as letting kids watch *Tokyo Drift* and expecting it to teach them how to drive. It makes zero sense.

We must resist against both the backward way society demonizes sexuality and the infiltration of porn as education by obtaining the knowledge we need to enjoy sex to its fullest extent (and have it safely). We can only do that by talking about it, writing about it, and actively pursuing sexually fulfilled lives. We must resist, and we must persist.

What am I even getting at with all of this? The message is simple, really. We have to take back control and educate ourselves.

We have to educate young people. We need to demand better from our media. We have to stop listening to nonsense, and we have to reject being told what we should and should not think about human sexuality.

You do this through sex, having sex, not having sex, owning sex in whatever way makes you happy. And refusing to back down. You don't have to march on Washington. You don't need to become an activist. You don't have to donate a bunch of money. The smaller acts contribute to the larger cause. They count. They make the world a better place for women. Own your sexuality and you are a part of the resistance. Your sexual autonomy is resisting the creeping veil of regression. It is saying "Fuck you" to the GOP in a fundamental way.

As you move into the rest of this book, as you pick up useful lessons on cleaning sex toys, being kinky, sexting, learning about ethical non-monogamy, finding a partner, and living your sexy life, remember this: It doesn't matter if you're trying to fuck everyone or you're trying to fuck no one. Whether you're a massive slut or not into sexual activity at all, your empowerment is still important. You are important.

Be sex-positive by being positive about your sexuality. Reject shame. *Sex-positive*, as defined by Dr. Dulcinea Pitagora, a sex therapist and founder of the project KinkDoctor, is about knowing yourself and being cool with yourself and doing what you want to do. It also means being cool with what other people want to do and empowering them to do that, even if it's different from what someone else would want to do.

Have orgasms for all of us, baby! Come as you are!

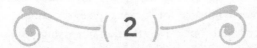

There Is No Wrong Way to Self-Explore

Before we get into embracing your sexy-ass self, we need to consider a crucial thing: Sexual empowerment means sexual empowerment for all. Not just white women. Not just straight women. Not just able-bodied women. Not just cis women. Everyone.

While we are empowering women to explore their sexuality, it is important that we offer a perspective for *all* women, from all backgrounds. You cannot have true female empowerment, true togetherness, without including women of all races, backgrounds, identities, and sexual preferences. If your feminism isn't intersectional, it isn't feminism. In order to own your sexuality and drive off shame and stigma, we need to join together and recognize that the struggle of one is the struggle of all of us. Together we are stronger than anything in the world.

Now, I'd be lying if I said writing this chapter wasn't a struggle for me. I am self-conscious as fuck writing about this stuff, in any capacity. Who the hell am I to write about the struggles of the black community? The gay community? The trans community? It felt like I was taking away a voice from the brave and amazing disenfranchised groups I so highly respect, admire, and appreciate. The imposter syndrome was kicking me in the cunt.

I'm a bisexual (but certainly straight-passing), white, middle-class, educated, able-bodied, cisgender woman. I looked at the outline I'd made for this chapter and thought, *Who the actual fuck are you, Gigi? Seriously.*

It gave me anxiety to even consider getting started, if I'm being honest. The fact is, even though I'm a white, privileged-as-fuck woman, and therefore it makes my writing about these issues quite ironic, they are still important and need to be talked about all the time, every day, no matter who you are. We need to fight for the rights of every woman, in every capacity, through every platform available to us.

Any book on female sexuality would be remiss if it failed to include all* women from all backgrounds and with a wide range of experiences. After all, if you're a woman seeking empowerment and decided to spend money on this book, you would be foolish not to want to educate yourself about groups of women whom you don't know much about.

When you write about issues that you haven't experienced (read: don't know jack shit about), it feels uncomfortable and problematic. Since I am not a part of every one of these groups, I decided to get insight from women who are. They can speak for themselves and obviously should. My intention is to be inclusive and to address some of the issues that women in minority groups face.

Thankfully, the amazing women I spoke to in this chapter were nothing short of gracious and forthcoming, offering insight into their unique struggles, experiences, and triumphs. No one told me to go

---

* *All* is definitely a strong word. But I tried my best.

fuck myself. Not one of them made me feel stupid or ignorant. Instead, they welcomed my questions and helped me along on this journey. Sexual empowerment doesn't get anywhere by alienating people or shutting someone out. It only moves forward when we move together. Women have such an incredible capacity for education, understanding, and empathy. And so much fucking resilience.

All of this matters because socially acceptable sexual expression is straight as fuck. It is white as fuck.

There is tangible, pervasive stigma surrounding groups of "other." I'm going to go over some terms that you may have never heard before. You might be thinking, *What the actual fuck does* intersectional *mean? Bisexuality doesn't always mean being equally attracted to both genders? I'm fucking confused.*

If you have heard these terms before, you're killing it! Snaps for you. It's still important to have a refresher. You can never be too educated, you know? In a dreary world of ignorance, the more you know, the better you'll be able to educate people who do not.

HETERONORMATIVE SEXUALITY: IF YOU LIKE PEEN, WE HEAR YOU; IF NOT, BYE

It is definitively heteronormative. Laura Warner and Michael Warner define *heteronormativity* as "the institutions, structures of understanding, and practical orientations that make heterosexuality seem not only coherent—that is, organized as a sexuality—but also privileged."* In other words, generalized, glamorized heteronormativity means

---

* Laura Warner and Michael Warner, "Sex in Public," *Critical Inquiry* 24 (1998).

that what we see in media, in public spaces, and in every other facet of life are basically all white and straight representations of sexuality, love, and relationships. In the media, the *majority* of television shows, books, and celebrity magazines celebrate white, opposite-sex couples. There are some exceptions, and they're growing but, by and large, heteronormativity reigns. The brilliant author and feminist icon Audre Lorde addressed heteronormativity and the contradictions of sexual and racial equality in her essay "Age, Race, Class, and Sex: Women Redefining Difference" in a way that truly encapsulates the suffocating straightness we see everywhere:

> Somewhere, on the edge of consciousness, there is what I call a mythical norm, which each one of us within our hearts knows "that is not me." In America, this norm is usually defined as white, thin, male, young, heterosexual, Christian, and financially secure. It is with this mythical norm that the trappings of power reside within this society. Those of us who stand outside that power often identify one way in which we are different, and we assume that to be the primary cause of all oppression, forgetting other distortions around difference, some of which we ourselves may be practicing. By and large within the women's movement today, white women focus upon their oppression as women and ignore differences of race, sexual preference, class, and age. There is a pretense to a homogeneity of experience, covered by the word *sisterhood* that does not in fact exist.

Lorde addresses the messages we see and consume, the ones that make anyone outside of the white, straight box feel intensely aware of their "otherness," leaving them with more questions than answers, further separated from the umbrella of female by the illumination of their differences. When all you see is a painted picture of the perfect Brad and Angie (RIP, though), Blake and Ryan, and so on, you grow to accept this as the norm, and to understand anything outside of it to be less desirable.

This "otherness" and often-resulting isolation women experience ranges from sexual identity, to gender identity, to race, to class. It is everywhere, the box so tiny we feel like we have to bend and break ourselves to fit the mold, or simply wither in being an outsider. The otherness keeps us separate, highly aware of the one or more ways we're different from other women.

Race has a huge impact on perceptions of sexuality. Writer Anita Little eloquently described the difference in cultural understanding of white female sexuality versus the sexuality of women of color in a 2016 *Ms. Magazine* blog post: "When you are a woman of color from a lower-class background, all your choices—especially ones concerning your body—are questioned and closely scrutinized. At the other end of the race and class spectrum, however, you get to claim you're just sexually liberated."

Sexual privilege and pleasure is a white thing, says popular culture. White men are the top rung of sexual privilege, but white women have sexual privilege over women of color, and white straight women have privilege over queer women. There are levels of privilege here. Even white people have privilege over other white people. Sexuality and an exploration of pleasure have been limited to the white, middle-class, privileged woman, the woman who we deem suitable to be sexually free and who we picture as the quintessential carefree, sexual woman. This picture of the liberated female we've been fed leaves out women with disabilities, trans women, queer women, women of color, and many others. Again, the strange thing is that I—a white, straight-passing, able-bodied woman—would be the one exploring these topics of inadequate representation in this chapter, but this only further illuminates the necessity to do so—I have this platform, right now, right here, and therefore it must be utilized.

Let's start with the first lesson I hope you take away from this chapter and with you as you move into the rest of this book: Who you are, how you identify, and how you see yourself has no bearing on your right to experience pleasure.

Anyone who tells you otherwise is a troll-y little liar. It doesn't matter how you identify or what your background is; if you are exploring your sexuality the way you want to, that is beautiful and amazing. Don't let anyone dim your shine.

While we're at it, don't let anyone dim the shine of others. Every single person deserves to self-express in whatever way they want to self-express (as long as you aren't hurting anyone else). Call people out on their slut-shamey, racist, homophobic bullshit—and call yourself out, if you need to.

THE STIGMA SURROUNDING WOMEN OF COLOR

In the interviews I conducted with women of color, nearly all paid homage to their experiences with some form of sexual shame, whether it be at home, at church, at school, at work, or with romantic partners.

Black women have long been both fetishized and sexually

shamed, a paradox that is both confusing and alarming.* As author Martha Hodes points out in *White Women, Black Men: Illicit Sex in the Nineteenth-Century South*, white men also took advantage of black female slaves, then blamed their crimes on the women's "hypersexuality." And this was just one small piece in the early fetishization of the black body in America. In "Black Actresses in American Films: A History and Critical Analysis of the Mammy/Maid Character," writer Valerie Coleman visualized the spectrum within the two extremes: aggressive, lascivious sexuality (not a thing, by the way), and the "mammy/maid" character, also known as the "good Christian Black woman." Just more boxes for black women to check.

I was nervous and excited to speak to Lidia Bonilla. She's a Hispanic sex tech entrepreneur and the founder of House of Plume, a line of gender-neutral, beautifully crafted boxes to house your sex toys. She says the company was born from equal parts passion project and her recognition that the market was missing luxury vestibules for sex toys. She used to be in finance but left to pursue more creative endeavors (i.e., sex toys). She's a cofounder of the Women of Sex Tech, a community of women in which I am deeply entrenched: a smattering of entrepreneurs, sex toy engineers, and ~~boss ladies~~ bosses.

I met with Lidia in a corner café on First Avenue and Second Street in New York City. She was wearing a maxi dress, fuchsia lipstick, her Afro bleached blond. She was my first interview. I had so many questions that I felt I had no right to ask. Luckily, she put my

---

* Black men are oversexualized, too; after the Civil War, some black men were falsely accused of the rape of white women. They were depicted as brutish, sexually insatiable beasts; dehumanizing caricatures that were and are extremely damaging to the black community.

nerves to rest. She assured me every question I had prepared was great, and she happily answered even the questions I had written off as too uncomfortable or ignorant.

Lidia told me that, to her, being sexually empowered means that you are comfortable in whatever choice you choose around sex. What matters is that whatever the choice is, it feels right no matter what anyone else says or believes. For women, that is something we (hopefully) evolve into as we get older. Unless your parents are open about sex from a young age, being sexually open and confident is difficult as a woman. Even then, shame and stigma fall outside of the home. Then, layering atop these realities, you add being a woman of color and, depending on your cultural background, different levels of religion and traditions.

Lidia didn't talk about sex with either of her parents growing up. They understand what she does for a living with House of Plume but don't really discuss it. She discovered her own sexuality through curiosity. "You know, I was always curious about sex. Because it is the one thing people didn't want to talk about. I was in church, and I remember hearing rumors about girls getting pregnant. I would sit there and guess who was having sex. 'She's having sex . . . yeah, she's having sex.'

"They were all about their pictures [at church]. I remember the picture of the prostitute. They had a depiction of her. She was lying down on her side. She had what looked like expensive garb, and she had one shoe hanging from her toe and was sultry. *Wow*, I thought, *she's so powerful*."

While Lidia had, in all likeliness, the opposite reaction to Mary Magdalene than her elders would have liked, she saw the raw electricity that lies in female sexuality . . . even if her little-girl self didn't know that at the time.

Lidia's upbringing didn't include a relationship with sexuality or sexual pleasure. She spoke about the same thing I gleaned in all my interviews: that pleasure of any kind is not something women of color feel they have the right to have. The more "privileged" you are, the more you have an access to pleasure. Not all WoC are working class, and they certainly aren't all immigrants by any means, but when you are new to America, a part of the working class trying to make ends meet, the conversation about pleasure is just not the same. Because it isn't the focus of your life. For many first-generation Americans, life isn't about leisure—it's about making a better life for your family. Lidia told me that her mom always put the focus on work and school: "We have to earn our keep in this country. I didn't learn to have a good time until after college. Pleasure is something I had to learn to do. For white women, it is their right or accepted."

I hopped on the phone with Cidney G. Green (whom we met in chapter 1) to talk about her experiences as a black, sexually empowered, all-around-kick-ass woman. I might have been out of my element and nervous about speaking with Lidia, but I was scared shitless to speak with Cidney. She is a no-nonsense kind of a woman with a nonexistent threshold for anyone's crap.

Cidney, as previously mentioned, is the creator of the "Pussy Over Pain" internet video. If you haven't seen it, google it. It is incredible.

Cidney grew up in rural Louisiana. She says her attitude around black female sexuality is nontraditional. She told me that black women are told that sex is bad, that it's dirty. They're taught that sex is the devil and you shouldn't do it. She says she told her mom when she started having sex and that her mom put her on birth control but that this was not the norm. "Black women are taught that men don't want a woman who loves sex. Everything you do has to be around getting a man, getting a husband, getting someone to love you," she says.

STI rates are higher in black women than they are in any other race or sex. According to the CDC, 65 percent of female HIV cases are within the black community.

In today's "progressive world," we view a black woman's sexuality as "victimized" or "deviant." If you're sexually active, you are either being used by some man—and that's very sad for you—or you're a whore. You're either a video girl or a Clair Huxtable. In Kimberly Springer's essay "Queering Black Female Heterosexuality," she points out how a black woman's sexual habits are a "crisis situation." Springer asserts that the "damned if you do, damned if you don't" view on black female sexuality leaves young black women without an outlet to discuss sex in an open and honest way. This is very similar to the sexual paradox white women face. As we know, we're all fucked. The big, defining difference is the ultrareligious thread that ties the black community together. It's not to say white people aren't hella into God (they are), but some parts of the black community revolve almost entirely around the church. It's how some community leaders keep people (especially women) in check.

"Black people are the most sexually repressed and the most religious," Cidney told me.

Extreme repression and a lack of representation contributes to the insulation of a community that develops its own unique identity outside of the whitewashed picture. They develop separate customs, traditions, and ways of relating to themselves and the world. Women of color lack representation in every facet of society—in the workforce, on television and in media, in leadership roles, and so on. I'm going to quote some stats on African American women specifically, but these are just to highlight the overarching whiteness we're dealing with here—a magnitude of scope that is undeniable.

Let me hit you with some fucked-up facts here. Workforce Alliance estimates that 21.4 percent of African American women had a college degree or higher in 2010, compared to 30 percent of white women. While white women make $0.78 to every man's $1 for the same work, black women make approximately $0.60, and Latina women make $0.53.

According to stats from American Progress, 13 percent of women in the United States are African American. According to the Workforce Alliance, in 2015, 57 percent of all professional jobs were held by women. Only 25 percent of tech jobs are held by women, of which 1 percent are held by Latina women, 5 percent by Asian women, and 3 percent by black women. As of 2017, of the ninety-eight women in Congress, only fourteen are African American.

Women of color need to be brought into the discussion about sexuality as often as possible because of these glaring inequalities in every facet of society. White women have to use their privilege as white women to elevate the people who are struggling. We all have to use whatever privilege we have, whatever amount it may be, to bring all people to equality.

This is no different when it comes to fucking. There should be no hierarchy of sexuality. Sex isn't white. "When you try to suppress sexuality in any way, you fuck yourself up. Sexuality is the most powerful emotion we have. It fucks you up in ways that I can't even understand. Getting some sex is the best thing you can get," Cidney says.

The body has a right to pleasure, and all sexual expression is natural and should be encouraged.

THE STIGMA SURROUNDING
QUEER SEXUALITY

I don't think there is a queer girl out there who hasn't felt unsure about herself at some point in her life. It comes with the territory.

I felt (and still feel) so weird about my identity as a bisexual woman. I only recently started calling myself bisexual to friends and family. After that, I opened myself up in my work. Why? Shame and stigma. Shame and stigma that we all feel in some capacity.

I feel like I'm not bi enough. Am I bi enough? I couldn't give a totally confident *"Yas!"* to that question even still. I date men the majority of the time. If I'm dating a man, does that make me less bi? There is an anxiety that comes with a fear of appropriating anyone else's identity. I don't want to claim queer culture if it's not mine to be a part of, and I don't always feel like it is that way for me. I know I'm not alone in these feelings. Many queer friends have expressed the same anxieties to me over the years.

As hard as it is to write about race, writing about queer identity is its own animal.

We live in a world that assumes straightness. It's the default. Race you physically see in most cases; sexual identity you don't. Everything is assumed heteronormative. You're a young woman, so you *must* be straight—until you're not. We don't look at a person and leave judgment at the door. We don't wait for a woman (or anyone) to "come out" as straight. That wouldn't happen. If you're not straight, it's on you to make that known. We're supposed to figure it out and come to complete self-realization without a single drop of help.

I'm apprehensive about the "bi thing" with men I'm dating. I feel more comfortable sharing this information with women. Why the fuck do I do that? I'm asking myself, seriously.

The messages queer women see are a jumbled mess of the following: *Bisexuality is a "phase." It's not valid.* This extends to all queer women, and often queerness in general. Queer women are constantly told their identities are up for debate and they don't really have a right to interject. *You must be confused. You must be questioning. If you're bi, you probably have not had the right peen yet. You'll get there. It's just a stop on the way to being with men, to being a wife and mother. Oh, you're gay? You must be ugly as hell and no guy wants to fuck you. Why do you want to be different so badly?*

With the exception of *The L Word*, there aren't that many television or movie characters for young lesbians and bisexual women to fantasize about. We've got *Orange Is the New Black*, *Transparent*, *Master of None*, and a few others. It's definitely getting better, but we still need to improve in representation. Straightness is still vastly the norm. If there is a "gay" or "queer" person on a show, they're usually played as the token LGBTQ person of the narrative—usually for laughs. *Modern Family*, for example, has a gay couple—the token gays of the show to add depth and pathos.

As we move toward a society that believes in acceptance and sexual fluidity (however excruciatingly slowly that transition may be), hopefully this lack of understanding, representation, and education won't be the case any longer. The Boy Scouts are starting to let non-cisgender boys be Cub Scouts, so if those fuckers can get on board, anything is possible, right?

I spoke with Claire Cavanah, author and cofounder of the feminist sex toy shop Babeland, to try to get a better grasp on being queer, sexually empowered, and female—and how these things intersect. It feels like a confusing combination sometimes. It fucks us up. Claire told me at the beginning of our interview that sexual pleasure is universal. Most people have had some pleasure, so there isn't really a prescription for how to experience sexuality. There is no right way or wrong way. Hell to the yeah.

This is so absurdly true. We have these white, heterosexual, binary boxes we assume everyone fits into, and it's completely fucking wrong. The general narrative has yet to reflect this fact, but it is there nonetheless.

I spent an entire evening smoking weed and drinking with my incredible literary agent, Ashley (Hi, Ashley!), and her group of friends. It was a Lesbian Party (yes, it was called that), and I was the only "straight" person there.

They welcomed me in and opened up about their experiences— what had brought them to New York City and a variety of different anecdotes about acceptance from family and sometimes ostracism from their respective communities. The whole night was ridiculously fun and interesting. While this group isn't representative of the entire queer community, it reflected (to me, at least) the different, complex, confusing journey that is figuring out who the fuck you are. One woman expressed the difficulty of growing up in an anti-gay Christian community in Texas; others felt different degrees of acceptance within their families, ranging from the tolerant to the welcoming with open arms. (According to 2013 data from the Pew Research Center, 39 percent of LGBTQ people feel rejected by family members at some point in their lives.)

One of the women I spoke to told me about her experience as both a queer woman and a woman of size; one told me that she'd been "straight" her whole life only to fall in love with a woman and discover that she was, in fact, gay.

Others I spoke to expressed their frustration with a lack of places to gather socially as gay women. A lack of public space for queer women is a pervasive problem. There are few places queer women can congregate and form community. Gay clubs, while marketed as being for all LGBTQ folk, cater drastically to gay men, leaving gay and queer women somewhat lost at sea while struggling to figure out who they are. Without a concrete space to find others like you, the struggle is even greater. Some of the women I spoke to expressed despair over their displacement within their own LGBTQ community, feeling left out where gay men seem more fully embraced. They felt discriminated against by the very people who were supposed to be family. One of the women told me a story about how she and some other queer friends went to a gay club only to be met with hostility by its patrons. Meanwhile, gay men have no problem frequenting bars meant for queer women. As one woman told me, there are essentially no spaces for queer women to hang out. New York City is crawling with clubs for gay men, but you can count the number of bars for lesbians on one hand.

This lack of community in adult life becomes only more destructive when there is no queer sex education to be found in the dismal arena of American sex education. When it comes to schooling, queer issues are rarely if ever discussed in a formal setting, leaving young queer folk with little to no information, save for a few Google searches. When who you are or who you might be is never addressed or acknowledged, how can you come to know yourself? How can you feel comfortable in your own skin? It is a scenario riddled with shame. If you don't even hear the word *lesbian,* how can you default to pride if you are a lesbian?

A 2017 study by trend forecasting agency J. Walter Thompson Innovation Group found that only 48 percent of thirteen- to twenty-year-olds (gen Z) identify as "exclusively heterosexual," compared to 65 percent of millennials. According to the CDC's 2017 Youth Risk Behavior Survey, schools that include gay-straight alliance groups for kids see a significant drop in bullying and teen suicide rates. Studies have shown that gay women experience the highest rates of bullying in school, putting them at greater risk for mental health issues than their heterosexual counterparts. This makes sense, as gay and queer girls deal with bullying on a variety of levels, including slut-shaming, queer shaming, as well as bullying based on their physical appearance.

Coming into your own identity takes time and exploration. You have to find your people and stop hanging out with judgmental assholes who make you feel like shit about yourself. It's a complicated and tumultuous journey for many women. With limited resources, finding your way forces you to rely heavily on community and self-education—objectively difficult feats for anyone.

In this same line of thinking, here are some things you shouldn't assume about queer sex.

1. All queer sex is risky.
Bullshit.
Queer sex is just as risky as heterosexual sex.

2. Bisexuality doesn't exist.
Bullshit.
Bisexuality is valid. You are valid. Your experiences are valid. A 2017 study, backed by BBC, of three

thousand Brits found that one-third of young people identify as bisexual. I'm still grappling, too. Many of us are. You are seen, bb.

3. One person is the top and the other is the bottom.
Bullshit.

People can be all kinds of things. You can be a top with one person and a bottom with another. You can be a top today and not tomorrow. It doesn't fucking matter because you get to be whomever the fuck you want.

4. One person is traditionally masculine of center, where the other is generally femme of center.
Bullshit.

You can dress however you want and be attracted to whomever you want. You don't have to dress a certain way to attract a certain type of person.

We need to work together to bridge gaps of misunderstanding about all things queer so that we can all come together to be better informed. Mal Harrison, the director for the Center for Erotic Intelligence and my dear, dope-ass friend, told me, "The best thing we can do is talk about it. And, it's to say, 'I'm gonna ask you a sensitive question, and if this offends you, I apologize, but that isn't what I mean at all.'"

No more ignorance, only erotic intelligence, conversation, and compassion.

ACKNOWLEDGING TRANS IDENTITY IN A SOCIETY THAT ACTS LIKE ASSHOLES ABOUT IT

I'm going to briefly touch on trans women because they have as much place in this book as all other women. Honestly, I didn't know that much about trans women or the trans community before writing this book. I'm sure my information is still lacking. Regardless, trans women have a place in sexual freedom and always will.

Having sex with a trans woman shouldn't be different from having sex with anyone else. This is the main point I gleaned from my interview with Zil, a trans activist and nurse who works with trans patients at Mount Sinai Hospital in New York. Sex is about figuring out what feels good and moving on from there.

To Zil, the definition of sexual empowerment is knowing what feels good and having the agency to ask for it.

When it comes to being trans, it's a journey of figuring out who you are, coming into that identity, and growing from there. Zil told me there is a whole debate about whether or not trans women are obligated to tell people if they're trans before they have sex with that person. There is such a fear and stigma around being trans and interacting with trans people. People have been murdered for being trans when someone finds out about it. The Human Rights Campaign estimates that at least twenty-three trans people were killed in the United States in 2017 alone.

There are so many questions about safety, and it's so hard to be empowered, Zil told me. It's not trans women's fault that sexual empowerment is so hard for them—it's society's fault, and it's a question about social acceptance. While there are many organ-izations that are working to allow trans women social acceptance, it takes people getting their shit together.

Gender identity and sexuality are two different things. The Human Rights Campaign has a helpful glossary for this, covering definitions and clarifications. There are questions, and we should ask them, even if it makes us feel uncool or ignorant. There is room for fluid and varied sexualities. Just because someone is trans doesn't mean they're straight. Just because someone is trans doesn't mean they are queer.

THE MYTH OF THE ACE

I don't know if you've wondered about this yet, but you should: the whole idea of asexuality and how it fits into this story of sexual empowerment. It is the myth of the ace: You're not sexually em-powered if you don't want to have sex.*

First of all, what exactly does it mean to be asexual?

Asexuality (*ace* for short) refers to someone who doesn't have feelings of sexual attraction. Ace people can have libidos (the de-gree of which varies from person to person), but sexual attraction isn't present. Sources have varied on the number of asexual people there are in the world, but according to *The Journal of Sexual Re-search*, it's generally believed that about 1 percent of the world's

---

* An aside: I'm not a scholar (on any of the subjects in this chapter) so I'm just briefly touching on them. There are so many incredible, inspiring, informative books out there on all these subjects, from gender theory, to asexuality, to women of color. Go read those books, too.

population is asexual—which may sound like a small amount, but is still about 77 million people in the world.

In her book *The Invisible Orientation: An Introduction to Asexuality*, author Julia Sondra Decker asks anyone questioning whether they are asexual to answer the following questions: "Are you sexually attracted to other people? Do you feel the need to make sex a part of your life? Do you have a desire to introduce sexual activities into your relationships?" Decker points out that asexuality is something you have to figure out yourself, and no doctor or expert can diagnose you.

There is a full spectrum of asexuality. Demi versions do exist—for instance, the need to have emotional intimacy to form a sexual attraction. There are many possible sexual orientations that fall in the ace spectrum.

You might be scratching your mons pubis and wondering what the actual hell this means. Well, I hate to break it to you, but sexuality is complicated as fuck. Ace people still masturbate. Not all of them, but some certainly do. I've heard it described as varying from "scratching an itch" to being really horny, just not in the way someone who experiences sexual feeling feels horny.

There are ace individuals who are repulsed by the idea of sex, and there are ace people who aren't. Some are fine with having sex, even if they don't have sexual feelings. Some are not down with that shit at all. Just because someone is asexual doesn't mean they don't deserve a full, pleasure-based, accurate sexual education. Even if an asexual person never uses the tools and information, they still need to know about it as much as anyone else.

The point is, this shit is complex, and we have no right to write off anyone or their feelings. Because frankly, it's not our fucking business how someone expresses, feels about, or enjoys or does not enjoy their sexuality.

I spoke to a woman named Serena (not her real name) about her identity as asexual. She told me she first understood her identity when she discovered the Kinsey Scale (which measures sexual feelings on a gradient scale from 0 to 6 and X) and found her sexuality fell on the far spectrum (a Kinsey X, meaning no sexual attraction). At the time, she had no idea that asexuality was a valid form of sexual identity. There is still very little information available around asexuality, and there is even an organization devoted to raising visibility: the Asexual Visibility and Education Network. Nonetheless, it still often falls outside of the scope of general understanding.

Asexuality is kind of a mindfuck if you're just encountering it. It took a lot of reading, interviewing, and research to get my brain around it. In my opinion, which is clearly gospel, it's the perfect example of how fluid sexual identity really is. You can be homoromantic and asexual, meaning you have emotional feelings for the same sex, but not sexual feelings. You can be heteroromantic and asexual, meaning the same thing only you have emotional feelings for the opposite sex. It's confusing stuff, but that doesn't mean it is invalid, wrong, or "less than."

Ace women (and men) experience similar queer discrimination, wherein they're told that they must have missed something or must be broken somehow. To not like sex is weird and they should be embarrassed. This invalidates their entire identity, and it is fucked. Some people don't have sexual feelings for other people.

You don't have to have sex to be sexually empowered. Sexual empowerment means having agency and control over what you do or not do with your body. It means being a human person.

Even if you don't want to go out and fuck everyone, that's dope. There is nothing wrong with that. You're not "left out" of the slut club because you don't want to have sex or are repulsed by the idea of having sex.

If you don't want to have sex, that is a form of sexual empowerment. You have the right to your own body and to do whatever the fuck you want with it. Whether that means having sex or not having sex is up to you.

This applies to everyone of all identities, so listen up: You don't have to have casual sex to be empowered. Empowerment means owning your body and your sexuality and not answering to anyone else's bullshit.

So let's get it fucking straight. You can absolutely be sexually empowered and asexual. You can absolutely be sexually empowered and black, brown, white, or beige. You can absolutely be sexually empowered and disabled. You can absolutely be sexually empowered if you are gay, bi, queer, nonbinary, or trans.*

Now that we've covered all of the stigma and shame marginalized groups of women have to overcome in order to explore their agency in the world, let's talk about the fun shit: how fucking awesome it is to be who you are. There is so much joy in exploration. Being a sexual woman who embodies every facet of herself? That is *hot*. There is so much happiness to be found in embracing who you are and loving everything that makes you you. *You* are awesome, and being you is the coolest fucking thing in the world.

---

* And, before you get all up my ass, all variations therein. Be whoever the fuck you want, too.

When you are a repressed-ass motherfucker, ashamed of your identity or simply wishing you could be someone else, that blows. That sounds like a shitty way to be, doesn't it? It's possible that your own identities* are holding you back in ways you didn't even realize, and you should explore that as a part of your sexual liberation. Being authentically you is badass. It's intoxicating. What happens when you realize being who you are is the key to setting you free? The world becomes your bitch.

WHAT IT MEANS TO BE SEXUALLY LIBERATED FOR WOMEN WHO AREN'T STRAIGHT AND/OR WHITE

Being sexually liberated while also embracing and accepting your identity—whether that be as a queer woman, a gender-fluid person, a black woman, a Latina woman, a trans woman (or any number of combinations therein)—is, again, not something you can fit into a simple, tidy box. Human experiences are different for everyone, and how we choose to express ourselves is our own prerogative. It's confusing sometimes! There are times when I'm so attracted to women I think that I may have just switched sides entirely. There are other moments in my life where I'm quite convinced I might be straight. I'm a peen-hungry gal, what can I say? Being sexually liberated and in control of who I am and how I express myself means giving myself permission to feel and behave any way I want. It doesn't make me less queer. It doesn't make me less of a feminist.

---

* Or identities that are there, but you haven't figured out yet.

And it certainly doesn't make me less of a woman. And fuck anyone who says otherwise. They can kiss my perfect ass.

Being sexually empowered and proud of your identity/identities are not separate entities. They aren't always one and the same, but they are intrinsically connected. For Arielle Egozi, a kick-ass intersectional feminist activist and truly stunning Latina of Cuban and Guatemalan roots, finding her place in the world has been a challenging prospect. Arielle has a nose ring that reflects her coolness. She's one of those women who you want to be like but also want to be best friends with. She makes you proud to be female. She is vulnerable and raw in a way that not many have the ability to convey. *Genuine* is a word I'd use to describe her, but it doesn't even come close to encapsulating how fucking baller this woman is.

Arielle tells me that she's spent her entire life straddling identities, never quite fitting in. She is queer, Latina, and Jewish. She has honey-colored skin and green eyes. She's white-passing when she "needs to be." People have always tried to "place" her and box her in but have never been great at figuring out how to pin her down. All the euphemisms intended here, by the way.

Finding her way to sexual liberation has been a battle, one she's continuously fighting. She is embracing herself one step at a time, the way that so many of us are. Even someone as kick-ass as Arielle is on a personal journey. Keep that in mind. We are all just trying to figure shit out. "My body has been exoticized and objectified since before puberty. I learned to wear big shirts and win people over with my personality instead of my sexuality," she says. "I started writing and talking about my sexuality publicly mostly because I wanted to give others a space to grapple with their own self-perceptions and identities since I never had one. I realize now that I was also very much trying to find that space for myself. I've been taught that being skinny, white, and blond is sexy. I am none of those things. I am the dark side of sexy—the curves, the curls, the deep hair. The kind of sexy that makes men think it's okay to touch, because why else would it take up so much space? I've always been afraid to take up too much space, and now there is nothing that brings me greater pleasure. I am learning to be loud, to know what I want, to exist the way I need to."

This is goddess talk right here. You take up all the space you need to take up. Do your thing. Being sexually liberated means taking steps to own your shit, not changing it to suit someone else. Fuck that.

Sophie Saint Thomas, a sex journalist and bisexual femme diva, says that being herself has allowed her to craft a life wherein her feelings and desires match her experiences. Sophie is a very thin, undeniably sexy goth girl with bright fuchsia hair. She tells me over tea at the Bowery Hotel* that the color is called *Dragon Fruit*.

She says that for her, there is no hiding anymore, and that is freeing. When you try to make yourself into the smaller, simpler version of yourself, it makes you fucking boring. "There was a time in my life, during college in particular, when my life did not mirror how I felt. I tried to squish myself into a mold of what a 'normal' girl looked and acted like, in part because I was in a small town in North Carolina and wasn't comfortable in myself enough to come out and live my truth. Thankfully, I was able to move to a place and find community in New York City that let me live in a manner that

---

* We're fucking fancy, okay?

felt true to myself without judgment. There is a lot of privilege in that. I am attracted to all genders and sleep with people when there is a mutual attraction or interest, rather than when they seem like a partner that heteronormative society would approve of. I commit myself to someone when there is a deep love."

THE SPECIAL SAUCE? FINDING YOUR PEOPLE

This can be difficult, especially if you're from a small town. I'm not saying you should leave everything you know behind, but I can tell you that it makes being yourself a lot easier. I mean, seriously, how could it not? "I've known I was bi since I was a little girl but only came out eight years ago when I moved to New York," Sophie tells me. "Thankfully, there is an accepting and sex-positive community here, which helps me be a sexually liberated queer woman, but I suppose living as a proud sexually liberated queer woman just means being myself without fear." You get the love from people like you in places like New York, San Francisco, Chicago, and LA. Big cities have diverse communities.

Jenny,* one of the dynamic women from my agent's Lesbian Party, tells me that coming out has opened her eyes to a world of possibilities. It's made her hopeful in a way she wasn't before. "There are plenty of queers in the sea. It has taught me not to settle, because even though it may feel like lesbians are few and far between, I will find my person."

---

* Not her real name.

BEING YOURSELF MAKES YOUR ENTIRE LIFE BETTER, SEXIER, AND MORE LIVABLE—THAT'S A FACT

Look, when your family and friends aren't down with you being yourself or have told you that you need to act a certain way, whether that be "white" or "straight" or "normal"—that is really fucking damaging. The fear of being rejected holds so many women back. The thing is, being yourself is better. It is always better. It offers you a happier life in the end. Lisa,* another of the amazing ladies from the Lesbian Party, felt like she was broken and unlovable for a long time growing up. Now that's she's out, life has a whole new meaning. "I get to be with a woman! I get to wake up every day and love her—something I always dreamed about, and thought I would never have. That's the greatest reward of all."

Being open about who you are can be scary for your family. Arielle says it freaks her family out that she's so public about her sexuality. "I write and publish, and it makes my family uncomfortable and nervous. I keep writing and publishing because until sexuality is normalized, society isn't safe for all those that identify as women. I have two younger sisters, and I want them to have the tools and self-awareness no one ever taught me. There's no need to feel shame about our bodies, no need to feel shame about our desires."

Sometimes your family and/or community never gets to a place where they accept you. This is the case for Lisa. Her family isn't supportive of her identity, and it would be bullshit to say she doesn't

---

* Fake name alert!

still struggle with this. "I always want to convey to them that this is who I have always been. I am the same person I was before, just happier and truer to me."

If this is the case for you and your family is like, "Fuck no. We are not about that shit," there is no shame in that. The only person you have to answer to is yourself. Their prejudice is their problem. Always remember that. You may think pretending to be someone you're not, someone easier to digest, is for the best. It's not. I promise you it is not. You're their fucking kid, sister, aunt, friend, cousin, and they should accept you for who you are. If they can't do that, they are assholes.

It may sound trite to say that things do and will get better. But they do. Your life improves drastically when you stop giving a fuck what other people think of you and start living your life the way you want to live it. If you allow yourself to be weighed down by the opinions of others, you drown out the fantastic dynamic unicorn that is *you*.

As Sophie so poignantly puts it, "Being open about my identity made my life better because I no longer have to hide anything. When we hide things, they don't go away; they just live inside of us, twisting and turning. I was a closeted hot mess! Being open about my identity means I don't have to worry about hiding or faking the way I have sex, date, and love. I wish everywhere was as accepting as New York is. And personally and selfishly, it's just made my life better because now I date people that I'm actually sexually and personally compatible with, which means hot sex and true love."

Jenny tells me that being herself has changed everything. She now knows she can find love. "I no longer dread dating. Each first date holds a more exciting promise. At the very least, there is an initial attraction and physical intrigue." She says that when she dated men, she didn't have the same interest. She found herself falling into line, becoming someone she was supposed to be, rather than who she actually was. This is a suffocating feeling many women go through.

All women, even those who aren't suppressing their sexual, racial, or gender identity, are boxed in and held down by the shitstorm that is society. We don't need to make it harder for ourselves by giving in to this small-minded bullshit. To be further restrained has the potential to make you dead inside. "When I was younger, around fifteen or so, I watched a lot of lesbian porn in secret. I was so intrigued and turned on, and I subconsciously told myself that this is something I would have to live without trying for my entire life," Jenny says. This is not a way to live. This will not make you happy. You will never feel complete. Be. Your. Fucking. Sexy. Ass. Self.

Being yourself and loving who you are is a powerful tool. Being unabashedly whoever the fuck you are shows others struggling with their own identities how fucking awesome it is to be yourself. You're doing a small service to the tiny humans out there who feel as lost as you once did (or still do). As Jenny puts it, "Less peer pressure, less groupthink, less brainwashing."

Using whatever privilege you have to lift others up creates a movement toward a better future. We live in a patriarchal culture that wants to hold us back, and it's time to step up and step together to change some shit. If you are a woman, no matter what else you are, that is something worth fighting for. We are stronger as a united front. If 50 percent of the population says "Fuck you" to slut-shaming, subjugation, and the commoditization of our bodies, we will change the entire discourse around sexuality and what it means to be a woman with agency and control.

Let's be women who love ourselves, because in the immortal words of every single person on Instagram: *Women who love themselves love other women.*

The thing is, ladies, we are all human, and we all make mistakes. Many of those mistakes will probably be made while we are intoxicated. Now that we've established that all women have a right to sexual freedom, we should probably talk about the stupid shit you did while you were fucked up.

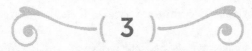

All the Stupid Shit You Did Last Night

Drinking is fun. That's why we all do it, right?

Alcohol makes stories. For so many of us, drinking is the anecdotal common denominator for all things college and early twenties. It is the fuel for every single memory we have (or don't have). Let's face reality; we are all insecure as fuck. We don't know what we're doing half the time, and the other half of the time, we're trying to look cool so people like us. Alcohol is readily available at every turn, and everyone wants you to drink so that they can feel better about drinking themselves. We go to bars to socialize, parties with ever-flowing wine and whiskey, clubs with bottle service. When you're freaking out about who you are, who you want to be, and how to get a life you actually enjoy living, alcohol is attractive.

No matter how many times you say that this isn't the case and you're being your "authentic self," remember all the times you got fucked up to have fun. Or, at the very least, when you got fucked up to help you have fun.

There is nothing to be ashamed of here. When you're searching for your identity, especially as a woman who is attempting to be sexually empowered, in control, and a badass in the work-place, it's extremely common to lean a little on your good friend prosecco.

This is a fact, and we all do it. We all get wasted, fuck random people, tongue-kiss strangers, fuck strangers, take our tops off, text our exes, and throw up in cabs. When you're new to the world of adulthood, whether it be college, postcollege, or both, you use alcohol or marijuana (or both) to calm your nerves. Maybe even some Adderall or cocaine to stay up, up, up while you're partying. Booze takes away your inhibitions and makes dealing with the inevitable anxieties that come with a newfound set of freedom and daunting responsibility possible and manageable. Hell, alcohol makes all of that pressure look small and easy to handle.

Since the presence of booze is almost a universal truth, there are likely some really messed-up things in your past that you need to acknowledge. These might be things you still feel truly ashamed of or traumatized or even victimized by. To embrace your sexuality without shame, you need to face, come to terms with, and move on from all the stupid shit you did while you were fucked up.

In my case, blackout drinking was a way of life for the better part of a decade. It was a way of life for my friends. We got along because we all liked to get fucked up. The booze was the glue that held us together.

When you get a little bit older, out of college and into the real world, the hard drinkers in your group start to dwindle. Eventually, if you don't get with the program, you find yourself getting hammered alone on a Tuesday night, watching *Sex and the City* reruns and chain-smoking Marlboro Reds.

Eventually (hopefully), you'll pull yourself out of this, realize drinking is only something you should be doing in social settings one or two nights a week max (and in public or with friends), and then move on with your life.

In the meantime, you should really get over the stupid shit you did when you were drunk.

A few years and several janky-ass New York apartments ago, I was lying in my very comfortable memory-foam bed (which was really just a mattress on the floor with a memory foam pad), doing literally nothing as usual, and my sister, Scarlett (or Scooter, as I call her), called me.

She was drowning in a hungover, nervous fit. You know the feeling: total panic over the hazy memories from the night before and a grueling, all-encompassing shame that spreads over you like a fog. The fucking worst.

Scarlett was panicking.

Apparently, she'd gotten drunk and slept with a coworker. At the time, she was an archaeological research assistant out in Arizona.*

"I'm really worried I fucked everything up by hooking up with Tim,† and now my time here is going to be even worse than it was going to be," she said. My sister is normally so nonchalant about everything, and here she was, acting like her deeply neurotic older sister, face-first down the shame spiral, freaking out over something minor.

---

* There is basically nothing to do in Arizona when you don't have a car. It is hella depressing. So, drunken mistakes are kind of part of the whole experience due to boredom.

† Who could have been named Jeff, or Todd, or Luke because who actually fucking cares?

Listening to this tale of woe, I was sucked back into memories of my party-girl past.

"Do you know how many guys I've fucked who I shouldn't have? *A fucking lot.* I have fucked *so many people* while wasted. And you know what? None of that shit matters now. I swear to you that you are literally fine."

I think I made her feel a bit better.

The thing I didn't say was this: What she did actually *was* stupid. She shouldn't have fucked her coworker, probably. It's kind of awkward. She does have to work with him every day. That's kind of logical, I guess.

It also wasn't the end of the world, and she needed to know that. We focus on these small, drunken incidents because the people we are when intoxicated are not (always) the people we are in real life. People say drunk words are sober truths. I have found this to be conclusively false. Drunk words are words we say to see the kind of damage we can do to our own lives. Who we are when we're wasted is the loudmouth douchebag who says every hurtful thing we can think of to stir the pot. We spent all day being wrapped up in this tiny, polite-as-shit box. When you get drunk, you get to say all the fucked-up things.

You have to accept your stupid, drunk-bitch self if you want to live your best fucking life.

That acceptance doesn't come without a little self-reflection and a bitter dose of reality. You have to figure out the root of your choices, the reasons behind your supposed fuck-ups. You need to distill down *why* you're doing something in order to truly understand it, accept that shit, and move on.

STEP 1: DETERMINE IF YOU'VE VEERED OFF INTO BEING A TOTAL FUCKGIRL

First things first: Are you a fuckgirl? She's basically the female equivalent of a fuckboy: narcissist, uses people, and toys with her romantic partners. She's a real piece of shit.

Now, a lot of this behavior is normal stuff. You're in your twenties (or thirties). You're young and living your life. You do stupid shit, but sometimes things change and the motivations go beyond dumb mistakes and shift into *Cuntasaurus rex* territory pretty fast. It's paramount that you can tell the difference between dicking around and actually being a dick.

Think about the following questions. Being able to answer honestly is a step closer to knowing yourself. And if you find you are indeed acting like a fuckgirl, *cut that shit out.*

Are you single because you love yourself, or are you single because you don't give a fuck about anyone?

If you're single and it's by choice, you're already on good footing. You can't really have a stable, healthy relationship with another person if you don't have a stable, healthy relationship with yourself. Are you *really* happy with yourself? Do you wake up every single day proud of the life you've built, satisfied with the relationships you've fostered, and confident in the girl who looks back at you in the mirror? Figure out the answer to this question. Even if the answer is yes, ask yourself this: How do you treat other people, especially the romantic partners you encounter? Are you on your own because you're just feeling this lifestyle, or are you alone because you fucking hate everyone else? Or are you alone because no one wants to date you because you're a raging cunt?

For a long time, I wanted nothing to do with boyfriends. I treated men like florals: in one season and out the next. They were a dime a dozen. If you're treating people like they are disposable, you are a fuckgirl.

Do you fuck a lot of people and are respectful to them after the fact, or do you fuck a lot of people and then ghost the fuck out of them?

Baby, go to bars every goddamn night if it makes you happy. Pick up the hot studs that catch your eye on the boardwalk. Get that phone number from that guy in line at the movies and fuck him later that night if you want to.

You do you. If that makes you happy, if that is what you enjoy doing, then rock the fuck on. I salute you.

But after these encounters—after these one-night stands and random hookups—are you being nice about it?

This isn't about catering to the male ego (never do that); it's about treating others how we would want to be treated: with respect. Don't kick someone out the minute you're finished fucking them.* Send them a nice "Had a good time" text the next day (even if you never want to see them again) and, in that same arena, don't lead someone on to think you want more than you do just because the attention feels dope. It does, but that's rude. We're all entitled to have fun, but we shouldn't aim to hurt anyone in the process.

---

* Unless you decided they'd go home afterward. In which case, it would be polite to offer to call them an Uber.

It's not that difficult to be polite. I mean, if you went out and the person was a total fuckwad and acted as such, then yeah, you can be a douche. But this is not the case most of the time. We're all just trying to have a good time and meet people.

Do you go on dates because you like someone, or do you go on dates because you're hungry?

You should *not* be going on dates to get free shit. Is free shit awesome? Yes. But this isn't chill. It's discourteous as fuck.

I'm not a super-ethical person. I've literally done so much fucked-up shit. And that's why I'm telling you this. If you're going on dates because you're hungry, you're just being a straight-up vapid cunt. I should know. I was that straight-up vapid cunt.

Get a second job or a better job, and pay for your own food. Are a lot of guys going on dates with you because they want to fuck you? Oh, yes, indeed. But be better than those guys. Go out with someone because you're feeling their vibe, not because you want to be fed. If they insist on paying—that's your call. Sometimes it's nice to be treated. Just remember—*you owe them nothing.* You should always be polite to people, but you do not owe sex to someone just because they bought you dinner.

Do you stay away from commitment because you love your carefree, adventurous life or because the fear of being hurt or giving up your control is too intense?

You usually end up acting like an asshole to avoid heartbreak. The line blurs between wanting to have fun and wanting to not get hurt.

If a guy wants to be your boyfriend and treats you well, are you saying no because you're not into him or because you're so scared that he'll fuck you over that you can't even muster the strength to take a leap of faith? It's pivotal you know the difference, and if you're a fuckgirl, *stop* what you are doing right now! You can't treat people like garbage. And you certainly can't treat yourself like garbage.

Being an asshole is not empowerment. Being an asshole is just being an asshole. You have to recognize your fuckgirl behaviors and truly accept that they are wrong. Now that we've determined whether or not you are acting like a fuckgirl (really, cut that shit out), we can move on to step 2.

STEP 2: ACCEPT THAT YOU *ARE* A STUPID, DRUNK BITCH (AND THAT'S OKAY)

If you find yourself on the tail end of yet another blackout, you're probably a stupid, drunk bitch. You've probably made an idiot of yourself. Accept it.

You will never mature and be the badass queen you are if you don't own up and accept the mistakes you made as a stupid, drunk bitch. And it's not even just when you're drunk. We all make mistakes regularly that we wish we could take back. We make them at work, at home, and with friends. We all fuck up.

This is the truth I've tried to hand over to the women in my life. My sister was a stupid, drunk bitch. That doesn't mean she isn't becoming a kick-ass feminist boss. She just fucked up one night. In the immortal words of the internet, "Chuck it in the Fuck-It Bucket and move on."

During our lengthy phone call (which kind of turned out to just be me talking about what a drunk slutzilla I am), I told Scarlett about this time I fucked some random Belgian (maybe?) guy in Barcelona because the guy I really wanted to bang was taking forever to get to the bar. After we were done (about three thrusts and a fake orgasm later), I took the condom off and, in my blacked-out state, tried to pull a Kobe and toss it in the trash can. It hit the window instead and slid down the glass in a gooey, sticky mess.

"That's disgusting," the guy said before putting his clothes on and leaving my room.

The next morning, the other guy wouldn't even look at me. Understandable—I'd been a huge cunt to him. He'd really liked me and had wanted to hang out with me, and I'd just gone ahead and fucked his friend. If a guy did that to me, I'd be pissed, too. It was not nice.

I was genuinely ashamed of my actions. I never saw either of those guys ever again. I can't even remember their names. I let them make me feel like a tremendous piece of shit when, in the grand scheme of things, none of it mattered. I remember it happening, of course. I learned from that experience. But it doesn't matter in terms of my long-term goals, earning potential, or anything else that actually holds bearing on my quality of life.

I was a stupid, drunk bitch, and like other stupid, drunk bitches before me, I got the fuck over it. You know why? Because of what I'm going to tell you next.

STEP 3: GAIN SOME FUCKING PERSPECTIVE

People don't care about what you do. People are way too self-centered to worry excessively about your personal choices. No one gives a fuck. I can promise you this.

They care only about their own lives. You are freaking out over how drunk you got last night; meanwhile, your friends are doing the exact same thing. And sure, you might have done something really tragic—like the time I passed out at my company's holiday party—but people get over it. It might be super not-at-all funny right now, but give it some time. It will add hilarious color to your life someday. We don't call these the *glory days* because they are particularly glorious. We call them the glory days because they provide the backdrop of story fodder for the rest of our lives.

STEP 4: FIGURE OUT WHO YOUR REAL FRIENDS ARE—BECAUSE YOU NEED THEM

Real friends hug you when you are hungover. Even if you tried to punch them in the face the night before. They know "drunk you" isn't you. If you want to find out who your real friends are, have a rage blackout and see who sticks around. (It works, but use with caution.)

One of my best friends is the blond version of me. We call her Sweet Dee (like in *It's Always Sunny in Philadelphia*), and the nickname truly holds up. God, I love that bitch. One night, we were at some Cinco de Mayo party in Brooklyn. I don't remember much of the night; I just remember at one point I wanted to leave and she didn't. I got *pissed*. I started screaming at her that her skin was going to look like a "leather couch" if she kept partying this hard. I know, ironic considering we were both chain-smoking and shithoused at this moment. She knew I was out of control. She called me an Uber, gave me her keys, and sent me home. The next day, we made up and moved on. I said I was sorry for being a raging asshole. She said it was okay. There was day drinking to do on a rooftop in Williamsburg, and we loved each other too much to stay mad. A good friend takes care of you when you're wasted. They always will.

Conversely, in an equally hammered, but less "happy ending" story, this one night in college, I got really wasted and said some pretty unforgivable things to my friend and roommate. He was super angry with me for a really long time. I apologized more times than I can remember. He didn't care and wouldn't let it go. In the end, it's probably for the best we aren't close friends anymore. He didn't want to accept the apology, and that is his right to do so. You gotta move on. I wish him all the best.

I can't sustain a meaningful friendship with someone who wants me to bask in my shame for all eternity. Friendships don't thrive in these conditions. They're like that succulent you bought at Costco that needs a lot of sunlight but a lot less water than you'd expect. You have to give a friendship what it needs or it will die.

A meaningful, long-lasting friendship will endure the tyranny of blacked-out, raucous bullshit. Close friends will hear you out and allow you to make amends after being a dickhole. If they don't, let them go. It doesn't make either of you a bad person. It just means you've grown out of each other and the friendship. Honestly, the blackout rage was likely a symptom of larger problems in the relationship anyway. Do you know how many times I've had friends say horrible things to me while blacked out? I know they're beating themselves up for it already. I don't need to see them wallow in it.

Your real friends won't do that to you. That's how you know when you have a true ride-or-die: That person will be there to pick you up even when you called him or her a "bad person and friend" while you were blacked out and struggling to stand. That person will forgive you and take care of you, even when you ruined the party and pissed off a bunch of folks.

And they'll always hold your hair back when you puke. Bonus points if they remember your bangs.

STEP 5: GET THE *FUCK* OVER IT

I know that processing the shame spiral is easier said than done. Trust me, *I know*. It's simple to say, "Get over it, champ!" But it is a hell of a lot harder to look at your bloated, smudged face in the morning and believe everything is going to be all right.

You're hungover. A hangover has the unique ability to really warp reality. You shake. Your heart races as the liquor drains from your body; you're sensitive to light and sound. You just filled your body with poisonous liquid. It happens. Your life isn't over. Go drink some goddamn Pedialyte, watch a movie, and chill the fuck out.

You have to remind yourself that this isn't the end of the world. Even if everyone is really mad at you for whatever it is you did, it will become little more than a funny story in the next few weeks. Remember? The glory days, (wo)man.

Am I saying we don't make life-altering mistakes when drunk? No, there are people who don't use condoms and wind up pregnant or with an STI. There are outliers here, but they are not the norm. That's what makes the shame spiral so interesting. It's the fear of these outlying mistakes that makes it all so incomprehensible. What if *this* time, you really did do something horribly bad? You probably didn't, but the existence of that minute possibility is enough to send you into a full-blown panic.

In the vast majority of cases, no one gives a fuck about what you did. It was no harm, no foul. And that's even if you *did* have one of those aforementioned fuck-ups—even if you did forget a condom or punch a cop in the face or whatever. You didn't die. You're here, right now. You've woken up, and life will go on.

I can't tell you how many times my friends have said things like, "Is everyone mad at me about last night?" or "Was I the worst?" or "I think I really fucked up this time."

Fuck, I don't even remember how many times *I've* fucked up, let alone my friends. And even if I did, I probably wouldn't care that much. People get drunk, and people do dumb shit.

You are not the only ass-clown out there. We are all enormous ass-clowns. After that night out, your friends are wrapped up in their own personal shame spirals.

Life is waiting for you to keep living it, not to keep stressing about it. Cheers to the next big mistake and living your best life.

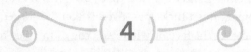

Stop Taking Other People's Shit

I jammed my headphones as deep into my ear cavities as nature would allow. "Yeah, and I'd like to bend that hot bitch from accounting over my desk and fuck her. She's such an uptight bitch. Stick up her ass." If I pushed the buds any farther, I'd have likely poked my brain.

Please, tell me this isn't happening. Fuck, this can't really be happening. People don't talk like this. This isn't real. It's a bit or something, right?

But no. It really was happening. It was a hot summer day in 2015, and I was stuck in my company elevator with none other than the Tenth-Floor Douchebags. My work wife had warned me about them. These dickmunchers had been causing a lot of problems for the women in the building since their estate financelawrealestate firm moved in two floors below my office. Running into them was the literal opposite of #blessed.

My work wife had told me a disturbing story a few days prior. She'd said that she was in the elevator with three other people from various floors. Two of them were women who didn't even work with the Douchebags. She said the aggressive vile things they were saying about women made her nauseous.

Who wants to deal with the pseudo–alpha male bullshit of some overgrown frat boy with a bone to pick with female kind? For fuck's sake, can't a person ride in a goddamn elevator without the fear of being aggressively harassed by a couple of dickwads?

It was sexual harassment. Every single day. In a Manhattan office building. In the ultra-progressive Flatiron District.

A few days after my work wife's traumatic interaction, I found myself crammed in the elevator with the Trash Squad themselves.

There were three men in the elevator with me. I was standing in the back, the three guys in the middle, and a woman in the front.

Two of the guys were pretending to grab the woman's ass and laughing hysterically. She didn't notice. She was wearing headphones.

I did nothing. I just stood there. And I let it happen. We reached the tenth floor, and all four of them got off. The woman was a coworker, maybe even their boss.

I was stunned. I felt like a traitor, a real asshole. I let a woman be borderline sexually assaulted and did nothing. It made me feel guilty and dirty. It made me feel like a fraud.

"You should report them," my manager told me. "That's really unacceptable."

But here's the thing: Who was I going to report them to? Who was I going to tell? The police? These fuckers didn't do anything illegal (technically).

I couldn't tell their bosses. I didn't even know who they were.

I couldn't tell the building managers. What could they do? Their job is to keep random people out, not monitor what happens in the elevator. I felt helpless. That's a shitty fucking feeling.

Here I am standing inside of an elevator, on my way to my job in liberal media where I work as a sex writer, in one of the most accepting cities in the world, and yet right in front of my eyes is blatant misogyny. You think you're in this insulated metropolis, but this male-centric fuckery happens everywhere. There is no escaping it.

What the fuck was I so afraid of? Being assaulted? Maybe. Being screamed at? Perhaps.

I know what it was, though, don't I? I was worried about getting in trouble. I was worried about making a scene, of disturbing the status quo. I didn't want to be blamed for making a big thing out of nothing. I didn't want to be called a narc-ass bitch.

This is what we women are all taught: Don't make waves. Don't rock the boat. Just stand by, look pretty, and be agreeable. *Be nice.*

Be nice. Be nice to someone who sexually harasses you. He's just complimenting you. You should be flattered. You should be happy when your coworker comments on your sweater. You should be fucking stoked when your work husband tries to make out with you at the office party. You should feel honored a man wants to talk to you, even though you are twelve and are walking to a gas station for a snack after school and a construction worker is telling you that you have nice legs. You should feel good that this guy asked you to suck his cock on the street, even though you are tired and just on your way to work at 8:30 a.m.

Fueled by rage and shame,* the next time I ran into the Tenth-Floor Douchebags, I was ready.

I was running a bit behind that morning, and a girl with brown hair and quiet eyes held the door for me. I didn't recognize her. Another girl was already inside the elevator. Directly behind me followed two men in their early to midthirties. They wore ill-fitting suits and clearly used hair product.

You could almost feel the aggression radiating off their bodies.

---

* Super-sexy combo. Highly recommend.

I immediately felt uncomfortable, a feeling most women are accustomed to. I stared straight ahead. Something was not right in this elevator. The two men exchanged some words. One guy updated the other about a "chick he was fucking."

"*Good morning, ladies,*" one of the men said. We ignored him. "*I said, good morning.*"

"Good morning," one of the girls whispered.

"There. That wasn't so hard. It's a really nice day, isn't it? That's a nice dress you have there." The girl smiled weakly and kept staring ahead. We stopped at the ninth floor, and both girls stepped out.

This wasn't going to fly with me anymore. I was worried that I might get physically assaulted, but I tried to remember that if that happened, these two fuckers would be headed to jail considering we were in the middle of a crowded building in which I worked (but, then again, who knows, right? Women are often not believed no matter what). As nervous and uncomfortable as I was, I knew I owed it to women everywhere to put a fucking end to this shit now.

"Actually. She doesn't have to speak to you, because she's a human fucking being. Fuck off," I said as strongly as I could.

I expected retort. I was ready to be cussed out. Instead, these two douchebags just looked stunned and confused. This truly might have been the first time anyone actually told them to fuck off, let alone a woman.

We arrived at their floor, and they stepped off. Neither of them said a word.

I still think about it, years later. This was one time where I stood up for women everywhere, but that doesn't mean I stand up every single time. It's not because I don't want to or think I should; it's not because I believe some assholes are more important than others. It's because not every situation has been or is going to be as contextually safe as an elevator with cameras in a building where I work. Not every person being a twat is someone I don't give a fuck about. Sometimes the person saying screwed-up things is someone close to you like your mom or sister or uncle or brother or coworker or boss. This stuff gets hairy. It gets confusing. It never stops being scary. I can say that with 100 percent certainty. It never stops being nerve-racking or uncomfortable or foreign.

You may be reading this, looking over the story of the Tenth-Floor Douchebags and thinking about how you've never stood up to a man like that. You may be thinking about how you've never stood up to anyone. That's really okay. I acknowledge you. I am no better than you. There is no reason to feel like a real piece of shit about that.

We're here, settled into these pages, because the problem of harassment, sexism, misogyny, and general shittiness is smothering. The problem exists. It's fine if you've never stood up for yourself before. It's perfectly all right if you take other people's shit sometimes. Maybe you have stood up for yourself and failed. Maybe you felt like an idiot. Maybe someone put you down and you had no response to combat them. That's a reality. It happens. We all get punched in the cunt once in a while—metaphorically, of course. Every single day is a struggle when the very structures of society put in place are designed to keep you the fuck down. Your initial reaction is to keep your mouth shut and go with whatever bullshit comes your way. This is how you've been mind-fucked into submission. We're going to learn how to make some changes, together. We're going to unlearn the code that has been integrated into our systems. Because fuck those systems.

HOW TO SAY "FUCK YOU"
TO SLUT-SHAMING ASSHOLES

The Tenth-Floor Douchebags are only one small example of the shit women put up with on a daily basis. There is no limit to what can happen. I read a piece in *The Huffington Post* the other day about women being catcalled and sexually harassed on the street while with their *children* or while visibly pregnant. What the actual fuck. Naturally, I had to ask my only friend with a baby about it. She tells me men still regularly lick their lips at her while she's pushing her daughter's stroller. That's so gnarly that it makes me nauseous. It's not that she isn't hot or that moms aren't hot. Obviously, moms are banging, but that doesn't mean anyone has a right to comment on their bodies. And fuckall if we're going to okay their being harassed in front of their babies.

There might be (read: definitely will be) some generalizations in this chapter. This is just a warning. The reason: The vast majority of the time, it's men who do this shit. When was the last time you had a woman catcall you in an aggressive and socially inappropriate manner? And when would that ever have been threatening to your physical well-being?

On that note, this chapter is about so much more than street harassment and verbal assaults in public; these kinds of interactions are often uniquely urban. But shitty people saying things exist everywhere, regardless of location, class, race, or background. Your boss could be a total dickwad, your dad might hand out microaggressions like they're free condoms at Planned Parenthood, your mom might think the only thing that makes you whole is a rich hubs, and your sister might be a judgmental, hurtful asshole.

The point is, people everywhere from every walk of life may put you down. Humans are kind of the worst. I know that sounds gloomy and pessimistic, but it's the truth. I'm not here to give you sugarcoated bullshit; this is not that kind of book. If you're looking for coddling, I'd suggest reading something else. If you're here to learn some shit, carry on. This is how we get fucked up by society, recognize we're being fucked up, rise above that shit, and then *resist*. I broke it down for you. You're welcome.

PART 1: TOXIC MASCULINITY AND THE HARD REALITIES WE NEED TO STOP HIDING FROM

Let's learn about *where* and from *whom* men learn to harass and harm women. Men aren't born sexist. They are made sexist. This isn't an inherited gene that comes with being male. There isn't some special sauce in the womb wherein one is infused with douchiness. It is a state of being that is crushed into wee boy brains from growing up in a culture that views men the way ours does. Toxic masculinity* is a hard stain to scrub (especially when our society gives fuckall about it), and men inherit sexist beliefs early on in their lives. Toxic masculinity tells young cis-male children that they are entitled to girls' attention and that girls' bodies are there for their use.

It isn't just us ladies that suffer from fucked-up gender norms, y'all. Boys get a shit deal, too. See, I don't fucking hate men at all.[†]

---

* If you're not familiar with the term, don't worry. I gotchu.

[†] By the way, I'm officially finished apologizing for sounding man-hating because fuck that shit.

I hate the way we've fucked up men. I'm not the first one to say this (obviously). Publications from *Salon* to *Bustle* to *The Guardian* have written prolifically on the festering disease that is toxic masculinity and how it affects all people of all genders. This epidemic is like that scary-as-fuck disease that spread and killed everyone in that movie *Contagion*: It's dangerous, it infects everything, and it's lethal.

Toxic masculinity places unreasonable standards on young boys and men, and these standards affect their relationships with women. When you tell a young boy not to cry, he begins to associate emotionality with femininity. I and most of the women I know have been called *crazy* (or something like it) by men who don't know how to recognize healthy emotional expression when they see it. We're called *clingy* for expressing our feelings by men who don't have the tools to do the same. We're told we're *bitches* or *cunts* if we stand up for ourselves because men have been taught that we are there for their consumption.

I want to explain to you, sexy reader, how this belief in female ownership and male entitlement can alter the course of someone's life forever. My life.

When I was in my early twenties, I had a friendship with a guy for a few months. It was one of those hot-burning friend-affairs where you spend every second together for a short period of time and grow "close" too quickly for it to be truly meaningful. He was a chubby guy of Middle Eastern heritage, and I thought we were just friends. Best friends, in fact. He seemed like a "nice guy." I know. Puke. At the time, I was newly dating my soon-to-be long-term partner.

For a long time, I tried to ignore the fact that when we went out drinking or hung out and were drinking at his apartment, he would make quite aggressive sexual advances toward me. I blamed myself. I'd tell myself I'd led him on and it was my fault. I told myself we were just friends and he understood that.

He was just drunk.

One night, I came out of a blacked-out haze with him on top of me, my pants off. My vagina was dry, and he couldn't get it in. I blacked out again.

Now, I fucking hate admitting this next part because it fills me with so much shame and regret: The following day, he brought up trying to have sex and how it didn't work. Instead of confronting him and saying that he had assaulted me and there was no way I could consent in that state, I told him that we couldn't hook up because his dick was so big. It wasn't. And it truly doesn't have any bearing on this story other than the fact that I made up an excuse to soothe his ego and brush my own sexual assault under the rug. I am still horrified that I said that. We stopped hanging out a few weeks following an evening after my best friend and roommate threw him out of my birthday party for groping me while I was only semiconscious. I never did confront the guy. I just ghosted him.

He felt entitled to my body and my attention. So entitled that he took advantage of me when I was intoxicated. I'm not even sure he realizes he raped me. That is what male entitlement does; it blinds us from reality.

Toxic masculinity teaches young men that women—no matter their expressed feelings—are ready and willing recipients of their advances. This can look like a male coworker getting butthurt when you aren't down to get a drink after office hours or as a male "friend" who tries to sleep with you after a night out while complaining about the "friend zone." Or, on the extreme end, and as with my experience, it can lead to sexual assault. According to an

AAU Climate Survey on Sexual Assault and Sexual Misconduct (2015), no fewer than 25 percent of women had been sexually assaulted in their college years. So you see, we all end up fucked here: the men who think this is okay in any way, and the women who are faced with unspeakable trauma.

In college, a friend of mine told me she'd been assaulted by a guy who lived in her dorm building. She remembered kissing him at a club. She woke up naked in her bed with him gone. She knew she'd had sex but had no recollection of the night before. She said that she'd tried to report it when she went to the school health clinic. When she explained what had happened, the nurse's only reply was, "Were you drunk? Because a lot of girls do things they regret when they're drunk." My friend said nothing else. She held on to that blame for many years before she ever told another soul. She didn't feel she had the right to do anything about it because she'd been drinking. She internalized her trauma the way most of us do.

PART 2: FUCK THESE HARMFUL BEHAVIORS. IT'S TIME TO SAY, *"YOU ARE UP FOR ELIMINATION."*

Because of all of this fucked-up messaging and bullshit, we're systematically reamed in the asshole when it comes time to interact with each other. Just look at street harassment and catcalling. *A question for men: Has hitting on a woman on the street and telling her she has nice tits ever worked for you? Has asking a random female-bodied person on the street to suck your dick ever resulted in a blow job?*

Seriously, I am asking. It is hard not to wonder where the actual fuck men learned that is beneficial to them to scream at us in public, on trains, on planes, in malls, out of cars, from windows, on the job, on their day off, on the way from the gym, while smoking a cigarette.

It has absolutely nothing to do with actually getting a woman to fuck him. It's about power. It's about making you feel small so that they can feel like a man. It is all due to toxic masculinity. Professor Terry Kupers defines toxic masculinity in his book *Toxic Masculinity as a Barrier to Mental Health Treatment in Prison* as such: "Toxic masculinity involves the need to aggressively compete and dominate others and encompasses the most problematic proclivities in men." These behaviors carried out by men are harmful to society and to women's mental and physical health. They make us afraid to walk in the street at night alone, holding our keys between our fingers like knives in case someone attacks. Men are told if they're not harassing women and womanizing and "slaying pussy," they aren't really men. If they aren't displaying dominance, women won't like them. And toxic masculinity is all about dominance; it's the definition of it. That message is completely fucked, and it damages self-esteem on both sides. The men become disrespectful assholes who think that acting like cunts will get them laid, and women wind up scared to be alone, ever.

My friend, we'll call her Jenny, was crossing the street in New York City. The little man turned white, meaning it was okay to walk. When she stepped into the sidewalk, the truck waiting at the light jolted forward. Alarmed and shocked, she hopped back onto the sidewalk. *He must not have seen me.* She attempted to cross again. Once more, the car leaped forward.

"What are you doing?" she screamed. "The light is red!"

The driver leaned out of the window and said, "I just wanted to see your face."

And that is what women face every single day. Men wanting to strike fear into us so that we remain complacent.

PART 3: MEDIA'S IDEAL WOMAN IS NOT THE WOMAN YOU WANT TO BE, YOU SEXY-ASS BITCH

We all need to stand up for ourselves. Women are constantly held down by the idea of being complacent and secondary to men. Even in a modern world where we're taught to follow our dreams and be anything we want to be, these messages still infiltrate our thoughts. They influence our interactions and behavior on a subconscious level that you might not even be aware of.

Misogynistic language of all kinds affects you. Remember "Baby Got Back" by Sir Mix-a-Lot in 1992? "Every Breath You Take" by The Police in 1983? "Your Body Is a Wonderland" in 2002 by John "Creepy as Shit" Mayer? Each of these mainstream songs sexualizes women, and it is fucking gross. These are songs that tell women that their only worth is rooted in their physical characteristics. It is dehumanizing and damaging. Straight-up, "Every Breath You Take" is about how it's completely okay for a dude to stalk you and follow your every move. But damn if it isn't catchy, right?

Other lyrics are even more sinister. Think of "Blurred Lines," the controversial and regularly discussed Robin Thicke song that had 2013 buzzing (and reached number one). The song implicitly encourages rape, crooning that "I know you want it" even when a woman may not, in fact, want it.

When I was at a middle school dance in seventh grade, the faculty allowed plenty of explicit music to be played for us tweens to dance to. While dancing with my friends, I looked to the right and saw one of my thirteen-year-old cohorts getting finger-banged to a Nelly song. She was sexualized and deprived of innocence because some older guy wanted to stick his fingers inside her body. I remember her looking really nervous about it, maybe even scared. When messages from the media tell us we're supposed to let boys touch us and do as they please, it becomes what we know.

Threats, harassment, and violence don't just take place on the street, and it doesn't have to be necessarily physically violent to break you down. Words do quite nicely, actually.

He doesn't mean it. *He's probably just trying to be nice. Maybe I should be flattered. He just likes things a certain way. He has certain preferences, and I just should go with it.*

This is what we tell ourselves to make all kinds of behavior okay. And it's completely fucked up. Ladies, you have to learn to trust your instincts and push away the brainwashing. You are conditioned to forgive men's transgressions. You have to remind yourself of this constantly. You have to force yourself to go against what you've been taught in order to claim your personal agency. To be a mothafuckin' *woman*, you have got to woman up.

I mean fuck. We are not playthings, here for the consumption of men. We are not these hyped-up tropes of femininity. We are human, aren't we? We screw, and curse, and fart, and exist in the world like everyone else. How can we possibly exist to our full potential under the terms that we be some lame, freakshow version of what it means to be a Woman? And for what? To please men? Come the fuck on. We need to all spend a little less time doing shit we hate to make someone love us and a lot more time loving ourselves.

In order to fight back, we need the tools to stand up for ourselves. This chapter will teach you some of those tools. But I'll be the first to say that you aren't just going to read a book and think,

I've got it! and suddenly be up in arms every time you witness some sexist bullshit. It's a struggle every single day that takes workable solutions to overcome. As I said, it doesn't stop being hard.

PART 4: YOU ARE CORDIALLY INVITED TO THE LEAGUE OF DIFFICULT WOMEN—WELCOME

Standing up for yourself doesn't mean being a dick for no reason. You don't need to insert yourself into every single situation you come across. Some interactions could compromise your safety or well-being. It may not serve you to scream in your father's face whenever he says something homophobic, sexist, or racist. What standing up for yourself means is seeing a wrong and not allowing it to happen. It means rejecting your internalized fear and not rolling over like a spineless twat muffin. It means doing something even if you are afraid. It sometimes means standing up to men who might be close to you.

My father is the best dude on the planet. He's basically my best friend. And for quite a while, I politely ignored the fact that he kind of liked Donald Trump.* I didn't say anything about it until, one day, he casually mentioned that he thought the wage gap wasn't real while we were in the car. My sister and I *lost our shit*.

It turned into this long, drawn-out, and exhausting conversation about right-wing thinking, conservative values, and a woman's place in the world. I didn't want to upset my dad or start a fight over his flawed thinking. He's always been 100 percent supportive

---

* He doesn't anymore. He thinks he's a moron.

of me, and I love him for it. I just told myself he was "of another time." When it came down to it, we had to talk about it and get it out in the open. There is no excuse for ignorance even when it's your adorable papa who sends you Amazon's top-rated erotica books to be helpful to your sex-writing career.

Men do not have the right to make you feel small just because they think they have an advantage. Men do not have the right to hit on you just because you exist. Men do not have the right to say things that are wrong just because they think there will be no consequences or clapback.

I understand why women often don't speak up. I mean, hell—as I said in my workplace anecdote earlier, even I find it tough. And there are many reasons we don't speak up. Here are some reasons we say nothing and feel like dipshits (usually, maybe):

1. We're scared that people won't like us.

If you're not liked and adored, then you're a piece of fucking whiny shit. Didn't you know? *You don't want to be that "angry" woman, do you? You don't. No one will be your friend. Also, look pretty. K, thanks.*

2. We're worried that the women who do what they're told will be the ones chosen as partners, wives, and mothers.

As we know, a woman's only value is in her ability to land a spouse and breed like hell. #CowLife.

3. We don't want to spoil our chances of finding a man by being too difficult.

Why wouldn't we? We've been told this is true. Look at

every Twitter troll on the internet: Their first insult to
a woman who speaks her mind is that she's ugly and
will die alone. No one will ever want a feminist, they
say. Feminism is designed to bring you down, they say.
Feminists are disgusting fat trolls who are only fuckable
with a bag over their heads.

4. We don't want a reputation of being "hard to handle."

Who would want to marry a woman who's "hard to
handle"? We need to take a step back because this shit
goes deeper than that. The idea that a woman can
even *be* "hard to handle" is fed to us by a social system
that fucking hates women. *Do you need to put in a lil'
work to make her happy or content in any way?* Hard
to handle. *Has an original thought?* Hard to handle.
Complicated and demanding schedule and/or life? Hard
to handle.

5. We don't want to be too "emotional."

Women are considered more emotional by men
because the Patriarchy works to suppress men's
emotions from a very early age. Because of this, men
seem to have no idea what a normal emotional range
looks like. We are so worried that a potential partner
won't want to be with us if we're complicated or
emotional. This just isn't the case. It is the Patriarchy that
has caused this failure in men to view women in this
way. We must reprogram humankind, one person at a
time.

PART 5: WHEN A WOMAN DECIDES SHE WANTS A MAN WHO DOESN'T SUCK TROVES OF ASS, SHE CAN RULE THE WORLD

Now, let's assume you're a woman who dates men or has friends who date men or family members who date men. Men with myopic views of the world want women with the emotional quotient of a toothpick. They cannot see outside of the structures they live within. Woke dudes can see beyond. Our vivacious personalities are what make women so amazing. Being a whole person with valid concerns and arguments and who wants to make those arguments is what makes you so incredible. It is what makes you human. And it should be fucking expected.

Admittedly, there are few woke guys out there, which blows. To all you ladies who only date men, my heart goes out to you in your time of need.

Assuming you date men in this instance, a real man—a mature, woke-ass man who understands toxic masculinity and its impact—can appreciate the best, real-as-shit qualities in a woman. What makes a man real isn't a fallback to ingrained misogyny; it isn't using words or actions to make women feel small; it isn't asserting authority to cradle his ego. It's treating a woman like a human fucking being. The fact that this is the bare minimum we should expect and don't is sad as shit. We're told to expect scraps of attention and affection—whatever someone is willing to give.

We don't even know what being treated well feels like, and when a dude acts remotely kind in any way, we're blown away. My sister and her girlfriend are still making fun of me for being so impressed with my most recent ex. He was—gasp—nice to me! He wanted to *be my boyfriend* without any hesitation. No hoops for me! He asked me to move in because he said he didn't want to live without me anymore! *Fucking swoon!!!!*

I would brag about how he brought me coffee in bed and bought me flowers. "Yeah, that's really normal shit in a relationship. I don't know why you're so excited," my sister would say. He was a great dude throughout our relationship in many ways, but the bar was set so low, how could he not be? I already expected so little, any kind gesture felt like it deserved a handwritten thank-you note and a blow job.

When it comes to relationships, it often takes an experience with being treated well to understand it. When you're conditioned to accept crap behavior, it becomes normalized. You adapt to your surroundings and internalize the messages.

It isn't until we're in a relationship with a person who treats us like we deserve to be treated that we finally know what it means to have a good partner. They are hard to find, but they're out there. It's easy to say that. It's simple for me to promise there are good people out there for us. Dating has steadily devolved into a steaming pile of dick pics, hookups, and ghosting—it's hard to keep up the faith. It's not easy to be an optimist in a pessimistic world. When you're fed a heaping dose of turd-covered douchecanoes on a daily basis, how do you keep your hope?

PART 6: STOP SHITTING ON OTHER WOMEN

Women, too, are affected by the socialized ways we box up men and women. Women are taught in tandem with men to hate each other.

Sayings like, "You're not like other girls"* and "You're so cool for a girl" are viewed as compliments. As if being a woman was itself something we need to overcome. We view other women as the enemy, a troop we need to prove we're better than in order to be found attractive.

The one activity that truly encapsulates this mode of thinking is shit-talking. We're encouraged to gossip, to talk about one another, to take our "friends" down a peg. We *love* to talk shit about other women. I do it sometimes without even realizing that what I'm doing is talking shit. Media encourages this behavior, it glamorizes it, polarizing women as crazy, bitchy, and catty. Look at *Mean Girls* and *Heathers,* look at *Clueless,* look at *Pretty Little Liars.* There are whole cinematic experiences devoted to how women treat other women like dog shit.

Women bring women down. We are our worst enemies. All of that bringing each other down a peg has left us at the fucking bottom. They talk about a girl's uneven eyebrows or comment on how fat Cindy from high school has gotten. We do this to make ourselves feel better. We want to be superior. We want to prove that we're better by tearing someone else down.

You know what I mean. You know when you've just broken up with someone and they're dating someone new? Have you ever gone through their social media pictures with your friends and said, "I'm so much prettier than she is. Look at that shitty weave. His loss!" Don't fuck around with me. We have all done this before. You feel better because the other woman isn't as hot. You're the prize. You win because she loses. Never mind that your ex is a raging asshole who sucks massive amounts of donkey dick.

Clinical psychologist and writer Noam Shpancer connects this

---

* First of all, women are amazing.

behavior to the influence of the Patriarchy, writing on Psychology-Today.com: "As women come to consider being prized by men their ultimate source of strength, worth, achievement and identity, they are compelled to battle other women for the prize."

I have a friend who regularly sends me photos of women she thinks are ugly. She always says we have to lift each other up, and then meanwhile, she sends me photos of girls with unacceptable buck teeth. She sends captions wherein she comments on their trashy clothes or the size of their nose. I don't respond. She keeps sending the photos. I don't respond. She keeps sending the photos. It's like a little dance wherein she tries to get me to engage with her meanness and I refuse to do so. I'm not saying I haven't been a catty-ass bitch before. I sure fucking have. But I'm making a conscious effort not to do this, ever.

As feminist women, we need to see this behavior as toxic to our cause.

REAL TALK FACT #1:

We need to stop pretending we don't engage in this behavior.

It doesn't make the nasty thing you say lose its nastiness by saying, "This is going to sound really terrible, but . . ." or "This is going to sound like I don't love other women, because I do, but . . ."

REAL TALK FACT #2:

By bringing another woman down, you're not elevating yourself.

You're destroying everything we're working hard for in the name of gender politics. If you let women be torn down and contribute to that destruction, you're one of the culprits. You're no better than a dude who tells you you're being "too emotional" if you raise awareness about something you're passionate about at work or a guy on the sidewalk who says, "Ugly bitch!" to you when you don't respond to his initial verbal come-ons.

REAL TALK FACT #3:

It doesn't make you look good or cool to do this.

It doesn't make you strong. It doesn't make you a better person or a more desirable woman. It makes you look extremely insecure. By focusing on the physical imperfections of another female, you're pointing out your own insecurities about yourself. When you call another woman ugly, you make yourself look ugly from the inside out. The saddest part is . . .

REAL TALK FACT #4:

It's completely transparent.

People know what you're doing. No one is fooled.

PART 7: SUPPORT YOUR LOCAL GIRL GANG

As Kyle Stephens stated during the sentencing of former USA Gymnastics team doctor Larry Nassar, "Little girls don't stay little forever. They grow into strong women that return to destroy your world." The times are changing, motherfucker.

Women are not taught that together we can rule the world.

Changes are actively being made by strong women who have had enough of this shit. Enter Shine Theory. Coined by Anna Friedman at *New York Magazine*'s *The Cut*: "When you meet a woman who is intimidatingly witty, stylish, beautiful, and professionally accomplished, befriend her. Surrounding yourself with the best people doesn't make you look worse by comparison. It makes you better."

Shine Theory posits that women have an unbridled power that is waiting to be unleashed. That women as a collective are unstoppable, fierce creatures who have the empathy, ferocity, and might to rule the world. There is enough shine out there for all of us. Lifting up another woman, brightening and reinforcing her light does not diminish yours; it makes you both shine bright as fuck. That is some Instagram-quote-level shit. We should all imbibe. Of course, this scares the shit out of men . . . which only makes it more fabulous.

A lot of men are scared of women as a collective. Men are terrified of what women can do when they're united. Woman power. It's what Inga Muscio riffed on in her soul work *Cunt* as the greatest terror of cunt-fearing men. They are terrified of the enormous sexual power women possess. Women together are completely unstoppable. It's no wonder the culture in which we live, the one that seeks to commoditize and shame us into submission, would be so afraid. Women are fucking strong. The vulva is life. The vagina is the epicenter of power. If they consider the enormous power that is a woman, they should be scared shitless.

We are only strong when we're united. If you want to be valued for more than just a small waist and big tits, you should start putting value on things other than the physical.

I have this incredible support network of women in my life. Some I've known for years, others only a few months. The women I've chosen as friends have my back no matter what. I can count on them. When I got my book deal, they celebrated me. They popped champagne and posted all over their social media that *their girl* was writing a book! When I was going through a breakup, they banded together to make sure I didn't feel alone. My cousin planned a fabulous birthday celebration for me. My best friend called me daily to remind me how fabulous I am.

My girl gang came from every corner of the internet and world to ground me, to allow me to lean on them when I was heartbroken and miserable. "You're a queen, girl! You are the *shit*," they'd tell me. Emails, phone calls, Facebook messages, Instagram DMs. I was loved and cared for. They let me know when I didn't know it myself. Everyone deserves this kind of support in their lives. Everyone should be a friend like that to their fellow women.

By this point in the book, I hope you've committed to standing up for other women rather than bringing them down to suit your own agenda. Women need to stand up for each other. If you see a woman being sexually harassed, and it's safe for you to say something, do so. If someone you love is going through some shit, be there for them. Stand up for each other. Hold each other the fuck up when the world would like to see you eat shit. By doing this, we can challenge hegemonic masculinity and the subordination of women as a whole. Let's fucking party, you sexy bitches.

Use Shine Theory to protect other women. Stand up to any person responsible for any shitty behavior. This isn't just about harassment, remember. It's about every form of put-down you can think of. Sure, street harassment is a huge issue, but I'm positive many more of you are dealing with crappy family members, misogynistic work environments, and horrible romantic partners who make you feel like shit about yourself. If more women stand up for each other, we can change the way men behave toward us.

Remember, when one of us shines our asses off, the rest of us shine even more brightly. Allowing someone to shine doesn't always mean verbally yelling at someone who wrongs your fellow woman. You can simply let your friend or fellow shero know that you're there for them if they need you. Remind the women in your life that they are not alone and if they need you, you'll be there for them. Send them reminders that they are fantastic. Lift them higher.

Now, you might be wondering: *How the F do I stand up for someone? I mean, I know I want to because women are* the shit, *but Mama needs some concrete info, ya dig?* I fucking *do* dig. Take a call to action in five easy steps. Let's fucking *do this.*

1. Assess the situation.

I got some badass advice from Debjani Roy, an activist for women's rights and trainer for Hollaback!, a nonprofit first founded in 2005 focused on teaching people how to respond to harassment. Additionally, I took two seminars on internet and street harassment, specifically on how to intervene as a bystander. That's right, bitches. I am a bona fide expert.*

Be aware of the possibility of escalation. Learning how to stand up for yourself or for someone else is the

---

* I am *not* an expert.

first step, and it is also the hardest. There have been
countless times when I saw something bad happen
and should have said something. I let my own fear hold
me back. It isn't always fear of violence, but fear of
ostracism. Often we say nothing for fear of becoming
the target of the anger. If you've done this before, you're
not alone. We all have forgone stepping in or stepping
up when we should have.

Roy says to look around and survey your
surroundings. This is particularly important in public
spaces like buses, trains, parks, or shops. Is it daytime?
Are there other people around? Does the person look
aggressive or intimidating? Do they look unstable? Ask
yourself these questions before you do anything.

2. If you don't want to respond to harassment . . .

Regardless of the circumstances, you don't need to
feel ashamed about it. You don't have to look back
on those experiences and drown yourself in guilt. Too
often we see something and do nothing about it. We
walk away with guilt on a foundational level. We want
to do something, but we don't know what to do in the
moment. I've been there.

3. Use a short line.

If you want to respond, keep it tight. Go for something
simple like, "That's not okay," or "That's disrespectful."
This works on the street, at home, and in the workforce.
Simply stating that the behavior is not acceptable in
a short and simple way can shut down an aggressor.

Not every time, but a lot of the time. If they get defensive, simply restate the fact: "I am telling you that is disrespectful, and it offends me."

4. Practice the lines.

Think about what you would want to say in an aggravated situation. It helps to know what you'd say. Be firm in what you're going to say. Stick to it. When someone is being aggressive toward you, you don't want the person to think this is an opening for a conversation. Make eye contact with the person. Take up as much physical space as possible. The whole point of verbally attacking someone is to make them feel small. Make yourself as big as you can while keeping a straight face. If you're on the street, keep it moving. If you're in the office, it's an old-fashioned stare-down.

My go-to trick in the workplace is to let the a-hole finish whatever dickbag thing he or she was saying while keeping a totally straight face. I then raise an eyebrow, let out a sort of surprised half-laugh, and say, "Yeah, this conversation is ridiculous and in no way worth my time." Then I walk away. That is a fucking power move.

5. Try to peace the fuck outta there.

If you are alone and this person is a stranger, try to get away from them as quickly as possible. Do not be afraid to dip into a store and ask for help. If you need to, run. Run like fucking hell. You do not want to give this bastard the chance to assault you. Ignore your instincts to be polite. But never do anything dangerous.

I was in a secure position with the Tenth-Floor
Douchebags. I was alone, but I was in my company
elevator. If they had assaulted me, I would have had the
police on their floor within five minutes. I think they
knew this.

There are all kinds of situations wherein you'll find you need to
stand up for yourself or someone else. Address each with an open
mind and a willingness to fuck shit up (metaphorically, eh, sometimes).

There are few main spaces wherein you'll likely have to de-
fend yourself, transpose an aggressor, and put a motherfucker in
their goddamn place. The main types are on the street, at work, at
home, and on the internet.

Type 1: Standing up for yourself
(and other women) on the street

It is possible to do this while being forceful and self-assured but
also remaining safe. Mal Harrison, director of the Center for Erotic
Intelligence, focuses on social intelligence and its importance
when understanding how to interact with people. She advises turning harassment around on the assailant in an attempt to shame
them—a tactic with which she's had great personal success: "Did
your mother teach you to speak to women like that?" is a line she
uses often. Mal demonstrated her tactic to a mutual friend, Bryony
Cole, the creator of the podcast *Future of Sex*. It worked. By posing
questions, a harasser cannot possibly answer without looking foolish. This helps turn the attention on his actions.

Bryony now says she has two lines at the ready: "Did your mother teach you to speak to women that way?" and something along the lines of "Do you think I'm going to just come over here and fuck you after you say something like that?" She finds it very empowering.

If a man fears being chewed out by every female he harasses, he'll be warier before doing it. If he knows that sexually harassing one woman will bring upon him the wrath of the whole female population, he won't want to step in that puddle of muck. We have the power to change the way we're treated, at least to some degree. It starts with taking care of our own. We are a tribe, and we need to start acting like it.

Roy stresses that safety is always most important: The threat of escalation can go from verbal harassment to violence. There is no perfect way to respond. If something works for you, that's great. The problem with shaming a person on the street who is saying gross or rude things to you is that there is a possibility that the shame could turn into physical aggression. You have to be aware that hostility and violence are unlikely, but a possibility nonetheless.

There will be plenty of times when getting in a guy's face is not a good idea. It can compromise your physical safety. Instead, try to get a message across with body language. Hold your head high and try to appear wholly unaffected by what this person is saying to you. Pretend you can't hear it, even if it is making you incredibly uncomfortable. More times than not, these experiences will only last a few seconds or minutes. Remember that this person is here to assert his dominance over you. He wants to make you feel fear. He gets off on feeling stronger than you. When a man (or any person) is putting himself into your space, denying any form of acknowledgment and keeping a straight face can be enough to defuse the action.

Type 2: Standing up at work

These techniques are not exclusive to street harassment. They are, in fact, quite fucking versatile. Just like that floral dress you make work with a sweater for fall. Only, you know, meaner. Use the same set of rules at work.

If someone is acting inappropriately toward you, you can call out that behavior. If you don't want to confront the person directly, find an ally. This may be your HR manager or coordinator. It is his or her job to protect you.

That being said, this doesn't always work out. I once worked at a start-up run by pseudo–alpha male assholes. The HR manager was their friend and was infamous for always being on their side, despite the countless times she claimed to be "for women." Another classic example of women fucking other women over. It was widely known in the office that you just didn't complain about sexual harassment to HR.

If this is the case for you, find another coworker you can talk to and seek advice from. Maybe it's your work wife. She can help you devise a plan to have this behavior taken care of in an appropriate way. Absolutely no one should get away with abusive behavior— not your boss, not your colleague, not your boyfriend, not your brother.

Type 3: Standing up to family, a.k.a.:

Your mom is being a psycho
Your uncle is drunk and telling you to "get back in the kitchen where women belong"

Your brother is bragging about cheating on girls
Fuck my life

Standing up to your family can be the hardest thing you do. They're your blood. Going against them is to go against everything you've been taught to believe. That is some fucked-up shit. But you know what? Some people are either toxic human beings in general or are acting toxic, and you need to put yourself first.

If someone you love, like, or respect is being a pile of turd nuggets, don't just roll over and take it. Tell him or her that you don't appreciate his or her tone. Suggest an alternative solution to their rude-ass word vomit.

When all else fails, which it probably will because family is fucking insane, walk the *fuck* away. Likewise, if you're a bystander to your sister getting shit on, don't pretend you don't see what is happening right in your face.

Type 4: The internet, where joy goes to die

The internet is the largest public space we have. You may feel somewhat safe behind a computer screen, but you're not. The anonymity the internet provides makes it a festering hellhole of harassment.

Though the internet can be a great place to "out" abusers, it also tends to nurture them like a petri dish of bacteria. We've got to chat about the darkness of the Web and how it plays an essential part as a catalyst for harassment. The internet is legitimately the place where decency and politeness go to die. It is the scum-sucking, bottom-feeding, neckbearded keyboard warriors' paradise.

Don't get me wrong. The internet is my lifeblood. I couldn't make money without the internet. Even with this understanding,

I can say with total confidence that the internet is also a terrible place. Being a woman on the internet is what I imagine being in public would be like if everyone wore masks and you could say whatever you wanted to anyone, without repercussions. It's easy to be brave and spew ridiculous, disgusting, cruel, awful things when you're hiding behind a screen and an extra-large soda. The anonymity the internet provides brings out many a troll's worst self.

The internet is the largest public space on earth, and it connects all of us. It is the world in a digital space.

I'm all for an open discussion and the plethora of differing opinions the internet can bring. It's a wonderful way to discuss controversial topics with people all over the globe.

Harassment is not the same as discussion or even a disagreement about ideas. Its intention is to cause harm. It's racist, sexist, violent, xenophobic, and discriminatory, and it's pervasive. According to the Pew Research Center (PRC) data from 2017, 41 percent of young people have been severely harassed online; 66 percent of U.S. adults have witnessed adult harassment; 18 percent of adults have faced severe online harassment.

People are the goddamn worst literally everywhere. I once pissed off members of the Men's Rights Activists/INCEL/Basement Dwellers Anonymous so badly that they sent a horde of internet trolls to attack me online. It was pretty sad, but also scary.

When you're a woman, this kind of shit comes from every angle. You don't escape it when you get home. The internet is right there, waiting for you. I'd know; I write about dicks and anal for a living.

The white nationalists (along with some depressingly insecure, racist, angry women) came for me on Twitter. I was at a club with some friends for a birthday party when I tweeted, "Watching white boys flirt is excruciatingly painful." Not that it matters, but have you seen a group of bros try to hit on women in clubs? Yikes. That is just objectively awkward and painful.

The white nationalists decided I couldn't be white myself; they wanted so badly for me to not be white in order to fuel their outrage that I became Jewish. I would happily be a part of the Jewish tribe if I were Jewish, but I am not Jewish. Being attacked by a group of wild, racist Nazis on the internet is always a joy. In this particular instance, it opened my eyes not only to how insane people are in general but how awful women can be to each other. At least 50 percent of the messages I received were from (extremely racist) women telling me I was just upset these bros weren't flirting with me and only wanted "pretty white girls."

Harassment doesn't just include words. It can also include images and violent video. It ranges from the unwanted and unauthorized distribution of personal pornographic images to videos depicting acts of violence or rape. The internet provides a landscape for a multimedia experience. This multimedia experience also applies to harassment. According to PRC, 10 percent of adults have been threatened online physically or sexually.

The worst it ever got for me was after I wrote about anal sex for *Teen Vogue*. I tried to keep the language as inclusive as possible. I wanted to deliver facts. The average age that a kid sees porn is around eight to ten; it made sense to me to provide something nonjudgmental and scientifically accurate to young people. I got a lot of great, positive feedback from publications like *The Chicago Tribune* and *The Huffington Post*. There was also some very fair criticism of the piece: I was so focused on explaining the practicalities of insertion and safety measures therein that I somehow didn't use the word *clitoris* in the article. As I'm sure you've surmised, I talk about the clitoris a lot, so this was a genuine error and one I readily acknowledge. See? Discussion of ideas.

Then there was the insane number of trolls who descended upon me. I was being smothered on every channel: Facebook, Twitter, email, Instagram. Moms in Middle America, and pretty much everywhere, were furious with me. I wasn't even aware that we were so backward that people would use the word *sodomy* to describe anal sex. It was a real eye-opener to how crazy, bigoted, and homophobic people are. One woman even burned the June edition of the magazine on video. Never mind that it was only published online. When you look to change the conversation or discuss anything that might be considered controversial, people will freak the fuck out.

FUCK, WAIT . . . WHAT *DO* YOU DO ON THE INTERNET?

If you see someone being harassed, you should do something. This does not in any way mean you should engage a troll. Trolls live for you to be upset. They want you to be mad at them. It gets their dicks hard.

Don't acknowledge these disgusting pigs. They aren't worth your anger. This isn't a rational person who wants to have a discussion about ideas. The only thing this person wants to do is say every vile thing he or she can think of to hurt you. Don't waste your breath, let alone your fingers.

Never read the comments from haters, block anyone who is harassing you, and report them. Lindy West describes the spiral of reading the comments in her book *Shrill* very succinctly. She says that looking at the comments is like going to a deli that only serves shit sandwiches. You keep going back hoping that this time it won't be a shit sandwich. All your friends have been to the same deli and tell you about the shit sandwiches, and yet you keep going back, hoping that this time it will be different and the sandwich you get will be the best you've ever had. You keep hoping that this time you'll see a wonderful comment or maybe a tweet from your favorite celebrity. Well, straight up, it's always the shit sandwich. The comments section is created for bored, lonely, basement-dwelling freaks to torment you. Just don't do it. It's not worth it. Nine times out of ten, it is complete and utter garbage. It is garbage stuffed inside of a dirty cheese-foot sock, lit on fire, and then stuffed up the butt of a person who hasn't taken a proper shit in four days.

Sometimes, the harassment is so intense that you can't do much about it. There are cases when you just have to ride it out and read as little of the hate speech as possible. It dies down. It always does. Ride it out. If trolls have one redeeming quality, it is their collective short attention spans.

Put a quality filter on your Twitter. It blocks out much of the noise from people sending acrimonious nonsense your way. Instagram has a feature where you can write in words you don't want to appear in your feed. I blocked the word *pedophile* and *pedo* after AnalGate, and the trolls took to spelling it in all kinds of creative ways. It was kind of impressive, but again, sad.

If there is one thing you should remember when the trolls descend, it's that these losers are so bored and so thoroughly unfulfilled that they are spending their free time (of which they have *much*) harassing women on the internet. You don't really get lamer than that.

You can't let the internet trolls get you down. You absolutely cannot stop doing what you're doing. Do not ever stop writing, tweeting, Instagramming, and being yourself. You should feel (a very, very small amount of) pity for trolls. They have no lives. This is literally the only thing in life that brings them a flicker of happiness. Trying to dehumanize and shame women on the internet behind the safety of their screens is the *only* thing they have in life. Will this make having horrible things said to you bounce off you like rubber on glue? Probably not, but it helps to know someone has your back.

FIGHT THE ASSHOLES
UNTIL YOUR DYING DAY

On that note, Roy says we need to recognize the emotional impact online harassment has on people. Most people experience harassment before the age of seventeen. Many women experience it around thirteen or fourteen. Whether we want to say it out loud or not, it makes us smaller, and it makes us inherently afraid. It changes the parameters for where you can be, what you can wear, and who you can be. It can impact the trajectory of a woman's entire life.

We have to call out that impact and recognize it. We can say, "Just be stronger," or "Just ignore it," to women, but that takes away from the experience. It invalidates a woman's feelings of fear. We all want to feel like we're not alone. If we can come together and realize that we've all had these experiences and witnessed these experiences, we can work to change the cultural narrative.

You can't go out without a fight. That doesn't mean you have to get in anyone's face; it means you have to help in some way. If you do nothing, you'll wind up full of regrets. It's just a fact of life. You really will become the complacent female that society so desperately wants you to be.

You deserve to be treated like an equal. This means having the *right* to go to work, the store, or on public transportation without the fear of sexual harassment. This means having the *right* to tell a man to kindly leave you the fuck alone without fear.

Stop worrying about what other people think of you. Stop hiding from this treatment. You can't kick ass if you're too wrapped up inside your own head to make moves. Don't let the bad guys win.

Remember, harassment is never your fault. You are not responsible for the way someone behaves toward you. Roy tells the women she works with, and women everywhere, that they are not alone, and she wants to ensure women that in her work, people have all kinds of reactions during intense situations.

Your sexual openness and your freedom will only get stronger the more people hate on you and the more you persist in your endeavors, whatever they may be. The more they slut-shame, the more you should slut it *up*. The more people tell you to stop, the harder you have to push. You have the power here. Anyone who makes you feel badly for enjoying yourself and enjoying your body is a piece of shit.

Taking back your strength means fostering the personal confidence and self-love to stand up against people who want to bring you down. People will try to use your sexuality and freedom to control you. They will always have something negative to say, no matter what you do. Never let them be the reason you give up. Never let someone tell you what you should be doing with your body, and fuck anyone who makes you feel unsafe.

It's a long and slow process. It takes time, practice, and patience.

Don't be afraid to be afraid; use fear to help you make a difference. There will be days when you feel so strong and so good about yourself. You'll feel like you can conquer the world. There will also be days when you feel low as fuck; days when you can't even face another dickbag human getting in your face. Part of growing up and growing into your skin is recognizing that there is no final destination. There is no ultimate enlightenment. It's a winding road full of ups and downs. It's called being human.

Tell yourself that no woman deserves to feel alone. You are not alone. You'll never be alone. Harassment is inexcusable. Misogyny is inexcusable. We need to stand together in order to change collective attitudes and behavior. It starts with knowing you are a badass and never succumbing to the unkindness and harshness of those who choose to harass. It starts with having the guts to stand up for each other and being there to lend a supportive arm.

You are a sexual being, and you should be proud of that. You know what else the internet is good for? Giving you information. You know what else the internet sucks at? Giving you the right information.

Since you're a hot-ass woman with a libido, who is not taking anyone's shit, let's talk about STIs. Empowerment is having control over your body and its safety, no matter what.

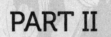

PART II

Living Your Sexy AF Life

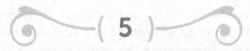

STIs and the Real Shit You Need to Know

This chapter is not going to be some bullshit where I pretend to be an ob-gyn with my mythical medical license from the University of My Opinion. I'm here to give you the lowdown on STIs, because there is some real shit you need to know and I, your agony aunt, am going to tell you about it. I'm someone with personal experience and an honorary degree in doing stupid shit.

When it comes to STIs, there is *so* much missing and false information out there that we need to sift through. Without information, you can't possibly protect yourself and your body.

There's nothing wrong with having a ton of sex, but if you're doing it without knowing the facts, you'll wind up on antibiotics or stuck with something for life. Herpes is not sexy. No person ever said, "You know what I find so insanely hot? Inflamed genital sores dripping with fetid pus."

Even I, a person who *does* know a lot about STIs and who always preaches about condoms and safe sex, am not impervious to the siren call of being a hedonistic dumbass.

When my phone started ringing, I was surfing the internet at my first real, adult job. That was the entirety of my responsibility in a nutshell: to surf the internet and look for trending news stories that our news writers would mock up. No writing, just net-surfing all day long: an endless flow of Kim Kardashian's ass and the latest cosmetic surgery D-list celebs had undergone that week.

I picked up the phone right there at my desk, a foot away from a copy editor in our open-floor, millennial office.

"Hi, Miss Engle? This is your doctor's office. We have the results from your recent STI screening. Is now a good time to talk?"

They don't call if it's good. I knew that much. Our start-up office space was too small for conference rooms, and getting outside would take too long, so I parked in the hallway, slumping against the crumbling plaster.

"It appears you've tested positive for chlamydia."

I froze momentarily, my heart immediately falling into my butt. I felt sick to my stomach and for a moment thought I might puke. The nurse explained that this was a very treatable infection. She asked about my current sexual partners. I told her I was in a committed relationship. I could hear the doubtful pause, like she didn't think I could be monogamous if I had chlamydia. Maybe her judgment was all in my head. Maybe I was just judging myself.

My mind was flooded with every bit of information I had ever heard or read about chlamydia. The voice that escaped my mouth was not my own; it was some little-girl, baby voice I didn't recognize: "What else do I need to know? Is there a way I can reinfect myself? Like if I wear dirty underwear or pants I've worn without washing first?"

She sighed into the phone. "No. Just use condoms and you won't get reinfected."

I was twenty-three years old and pretty well informed about STIs. And yet here I was, asking a medical professional if I could get chlamydia by wearing dirty jeans. It was like I'd forgotten everything I thought I knew. STIs didn't feel real to me until that very moment.

I then had to tell my then-partner the news. With sweaty palms and near shit-my-pants fear, I told him I had an STI.

It's unclear who had the infection first, but I was relieved that instead of playing the blame game and instead of yelling at me or dumping me, my boyfriend came with me to the pharmacy to get the azithromycin. The nurse had called in a dose for both of us.

One dose of a medium-sized red pill.

And that was that. I was STI-free.

Confession time: I had been showing signs of what I assumed was a proneness to vaginal yeast infections for over two years before I tested positive for the big C. I treated the yeast infections with antifungals and probiotics; the symptoms would subside and then return the next time I had sex, wore a wet bathing suit, or spent too many hours sitting at my desk in tights.

Here is where I got fucked up: The itching, burning, and discharge associated with a yeast infection are also the symptoms of a chlamydia infection *and* a bacterial vaginosis infection. All the symptoms are itching, burning, a strange smell, and discharge.

I didn't test positive for chlamydia the previous year, but when I took that big dose of azithromycin, the symptoms of a yeast infection never reared their head again. It turns out I was walking around with a scorching case of bacterial vaginosis (and chlamydia) and treating the symptoms as if they were a fungal yeast infection. See, Auntie Gigi is just as behind in the game as everyone else.

For those of you who don't know, a yeast infection is an uncomfortable infection of the vagina caused by an overgrowth of the fungus candida. Symptoms include itching, burning, soreness, pain during intercourse and/or urination, and vaginal discharge. The discharge is usually the consistency of cottage cheese. Isn't that lovely?

A yeast infection occurs for a variety of reasons. If you've been on antibiotics, they can wipe your vagina of its good, pH-balancing bacteria, causing an overgrowth of yeast. Yeast infections can also happen when your vagina is damp for a prolonged period, spurring an overgrowth of yeast and essentially turning your pussy into a bread bakery.

Professionals at Monistat (the company that makes my favorite fungal-fighting medication) say you should avoid being in wet bathing suits and anything that prevents your vagina from staying dry as much as possible. Otherwise, the balance of bacteria and pH in your hoo-ha will get thrown off, and you can and will get a yeast infection.

The only way to know for sure what you are dealing with is to be tested regularly.

Planned Parenthood advises having yearly screenings if you're in a monogamous relationship. According to the Centers for Disease Control and Prevention (CDC), 50–75 percent of chlamydia cases have no symptoms at all. The only way to be sure if you have something is to have a screening.

According to the CDC, chlamydia, when left untreated, can cause both serious harm to a woman's reproductive system and contribute to an ectopic pregnancy. When caught early, however, chla-mydia is not a big deal. It is basically a vagina cold, but if you don't get tested for it and it just goes untreated, you can damage your ovaries! Isn't that fun!?!

So don't be like me. If you're having sex with multiple part-ners, get tested every eight weeks. If you feel like there might be something—*anything*—going on in your nether regions, just go see a doctor. An aversion to a doctor's office is no reason to wind up with a lazy ovary or something even worse.

Now, before we get into STIs and how to protect yourself, let's start with some *very* important food for thought: Fuck anyone who shames you. STIs are not cause for public scorn and outrage, and anyone who acts otherwise is operating out of their own demented and fearful paradigm. Fuck them. If you *weren't* exclusive or you contracted the STI in the time before you met/became exclu-sive, your partner has no right to shame you. You made a fucking mistake. You're a human being. (The tiny asterisk on the anti-shame train is if you cheated on your partner and gave them an STI, then yes—this person has every right to be angry with you. That was a fucked-up thing to do. You'll learn from that experience, if that's the case.)

Anyway, back to the basics.

STD stands for *sexually transmitted disease*. *STI* stands for *sexu-ally transmitted infection*. So what is the difference, and when should you use each term?

We have to first define the difference between *disease* and *infec-tion*. A disease is an infection that develops into a chronic condi-tion and lasts over a long period of time. An infection is curable with medication, like the common cold or the clap (gonorrhea).

Not every person who is infected with an STI shows symptoms of the infection. Therefore, it never becomes a disease. A round of antibiotics will usually kill most of these infections. A disease is something ongoing—something you can treat but not cure (such as HIV). The sexual health community is moving away from using *STD* as the standard term, since most sexually transmitted "diseases" are actually *infections* that can be treated. Hence why we've started calling them *STIs*.

Are you with me so far? Essentially, *STD* is just not the right acronym for what we're dealing with, which are sexually transmitted infections.

An example: Most HPV infections will not develop into the disease called *cervical cancer*. The HPV virus usually clears up on its own and is therefore an infection.

We use the word *disease* only because we're used to stigmatizing sex and promiscuity. It's very damaging to a person's self-esteem to call him or her *diseased*. It makes people feel tainted, dirty, and unlovable when what they're dealing with is probably curable with a dose of azithromycin or something very similar.

While the majority of STD side effects disturb the lives of women, STI infections are equally distributed between men and women.

STIs *suck*, but we need to up the volume on education and turn down the sound on shame; there's a true need for the term *STI* and information around what it actually means.

We have to take the boogeyman out of STIs and replace it with facts. If we don't have the proper knowledge and don't educate young people about how their bodies work, how can we expect to curb the ever-growing STI rates in this country?

THE BIG EIGHT FACT SHEET

The CDC recognizes eight STIs as the most common and pervasive. So let's talk about the Big Eight. The more you know, the better equipped you will be to avoid being infected or infecting others.

If you've had an STI and been treated, you can still be infected again if you're exposed to someone who has it. You do not become immune to STIs after treatment. It's not the fucking chicken pox. Got it?

Here is what you need to know. Because when it comes to your health, now is not the time to fuck around.

Chlamydia

What it is: Chlamydia is a common bacterial infection.

Who it affects: Both men and women.* You can get chlamydia through vaginal, anal, or oral contact.

Symptoms: Burning, itching, discharge, bleeding between periods; 50–75 percent of those infected will not show symptoms.

How it's treated: Chlamydia is treated with a round of antibiotics, such as erythromycin or doxycycline. If your partner has been exposed, he or she should receive the same treatment. It is curable with antibiotics. You essentially take the same shit for a case of strep throat—only it's penicillin and you get to take

---

* Keep in mind, I'm using the terms *men* and *women* because that is the way medical information is presented. Hopefully one day soon, we will have good information for gender nonbinary, genderqueer people, and so on. But we're not there yet. Which blows.

it for, like, ten days. (Rolling my eyes into my asshole because everybody needs to fucking chill.)

Gonorrhea

What it is: Gonorrhea is a bacterial infection.

Who it affects: Both men and women. It is spread through sexual contact of any kind, including anal, oral, or vaginal. It can also be spread through contact with the urethra.

Symptoms: Pain while urinating, swollen testicles, yellow or green discharge.

How it's treated: According to the CDC, some strains of gonorrhea have become resistant to antibiotics and are therefore harder to cure. Because of its resistance, the CDC now recommends dual treatment for gonorrhea: a single dose of 250 milligrams of intramuscular ceftriaxone *and* 1 gram of azithromycin.

Herpes

What it is: Genital herpes is a virus caused by either of two different viruses: herpes simplex 1 and herpes simplex 2.

Who it affects: Both men and women can get the herpes virus. The CDC estimates that one in six adults between the ages of fourteen to forty-nine years old currently has the herpes virus. You can get the herpes virus by having unprotected anal, vaginal, or oral sex with someone who is infected. You're more likely to get it if the person is in an outbreak, but you can still contract the virus when the infected person is asymptomatic. You will not be tested for herpes on a standard STI panel. It is done through separate blood work and only when requested. The only time a doctor will suggest a herpes screening is if they expect infection, a.k.a. big-old tasty sores on your nether regions.

Symptoms: Contrary to what you might believe, most people who have genital herpes don't even know they do. People with the virus often mistake herpes sores for ingrown hairs or pimples. The first outbreak you have is usually the most severe and can be very painful. Outbreaks are not usually isolated and will likely continue to occur. Other symptoms include bleeding between periods and discharge. Genital herpes is called HSV-2. Herpes can also present as cold sores, the virus HSV-1. Yep, yep. Cool, cool, cool. Cold sores are herpes. If you have a cold sore and give oral sex, you can give your partner oral herpes on their genitals. Yay! So fun, right?

How it's treated: Herpes is not curable, but it is treated with daily antivirals to reduce outbreaks and the chances of passing the virus to sexual partners.

HPV

What it is: HPV stands for *human papillomavirus* and is one of the most complicated and hard-to-understand STIs there are. Even I'm still confused by HPV. There are more than 150 related HPV strains, forty of which can infect the genital area.

Who it affects: It can affect both men and women. HPV is the most common STI there is in the whole damn world. According to the CDC, nearly every single adult will have some form of HPV in his or her life. Over seventy-nine million people currently have HPV. I know: WTF. I had a cervical ablation in March of 2018 because I got such an aggressive strain, despite being vaccinated. My doctor had to put me under anesthesia in the hospital and use a fucking laser to remove all the abnormal cells. Bits of charred, yellow cervix expelled themselves from my vagina for six whole weeks. Hurray for HPV, said no person in the history of the universe. Fuck you, HPV.

Symptoms: Most people never show symptoms, and nine out of ten cases of HPV will clear up on their own within two years. The only way you'll know you have HPV is if you have an abnormal pap smear. Your gyno will then want to do a cervical biopsy to determine the strain. Legit, you will walk around la-la-la not knowing you have HPV. Some strains can cause cancer in the cervix, vagina, anus, and penis. Every year, HPV is responsible for more than forty-two thousand cases of cancer in the United States.

How it's treated: There is no cure for HPV, but most strains clear up on their own. Three doses of the HPV vaccine prevent most of the harmful, cancer-causing strains. There is no test for men, and it is not tested on a regular STI panel.

Hepatitis B

What it is: Hepatitis B is a liver infection caused by the hepatitis B virus.

Who it affects: Both men and women. Hepatitis B is transmitted when blood, semen, or any other bodily fluid is exchanged. You can pass it through sex or by sharing needles. Hepatitis B infections have drastically declined and affect fewer than five thousand Americans due to the hep B vaccination.

Symptoms: There are shitloads of signs you've been infected with hepatitis B, but the symptoms usually manifest like a terrible flu.

How it's treated: Hep B can become a chronic illness, but it's usually short-term. Only 2–6 percent of adults infected wind up with long-term hep B. There is no treatment for the infection itself. The best prevention is the hep B vaccine.

HIV

What it is: HIV stands for *human immunodeficiency virus.* It attacks the body's immune system through the T cells. Your T cells are the cells that protect your body from infection. When HIV kills them off, it makes it harder to fight off common infections, such as a cold or the flu. HIV becomes AIDS when your T cell count drops below two hundred cells per cubic millimeter.

Who it affects: HIV can be transmitted through sex or sharing needles. It can also be passed from an infected mother to her infant during delivery.

Symptoms: Flu-like symptoms will occur two to four weeks after infection.

How it's treated: There is no cure for HIV. If you're having sex with multiple partners, you should be on PrEP, a daily medication that helps stop the spread of HIV in the body. This does not mean condoms are not a thing. You *always* should use condoms (either internal or external). Even during blow jobs or cunnilingus.

Trichomoniasis

What it is: Trich is caused by a shitty little fucker called *Trichomonas vaginalis,* a protozoan parasite.

Who it affects: It affects both men and women. It's passed through vaginal sex or from vagina to vagina. For once, anal is the winner in this equation. Who knew?

Symptoms: Burning, itching, redness, and swelling of the junk. Seventy percent of those infected will not show symptoms.

How it's treated: It can be cured with a big-old dose of metronida-
zole or tinidazole.

Syphilis

What it is: The Syph is an STD that used to destroy people's nervous systems because there was no cure.

Who it affects: Men and women can both contract syphilis.

Symptoms: There are four stages of syphilis: primary, secondary,
latent, and tertiary. When infected, you'll experience sores on
the vagina, anus, and mouth as well as skin rashes. You must
have it treated within the first two stages. Otherwise, it may
be incurable.

How it's treated: Antibiotics can knock that fucker out in the primary and secondary stages.

Moral of the story: use condoms. Please. Get on PrEP if you want to be
extra safe. There is no "safe sex," but there is "safer sex."

Condoms are the worst. I get it. They are uncomfortable and
dry your pussy out like the Sahara Desert. It's also easy to think
that you won't be the one to pick up an STI. We think if our partner
tells us he or she was "just tested," that it makes it all right to forgo
a condom. But guess what? One in every three people has an STI.

Men, especially, may not even know that they have an STI.
That's right: If a man has HPV, for example, he doesn't even know
it. He won't even test positive for it, because a male test for HPV
doesn't exist! How about that? While about 40 percent of oral and
anal cancers are found in men, cervical cancer is much more common. According to CDC, 90 percent of cervical and anal cancers
are thought to be caused by HPV.

What's really absurd is the unconcerned way so many medical

professionals seem to treat HPV in general. Of those doctors I've spoken to personally, they often say that because so many cases of HPV wind up clearing themselves up, developing ways to inform people about their status would cause mass hysteria. It's reflective of the ways the medical community treats the testing of genital herpes. Since 12 percent of the population have HSV-2 (and so many more have HSV-1, or oral Herpes), testing for it on a regular STI panel would cause panic. Meanwhile the only way to know if a person has HPV is through a Pap smear, a test only female-bodied people can have. This inherently puts the responsibility of informing a partner about positive HPV status on women, creating yet another Blame Vortex in which to shame women for being "loose." A man may have HPV, but he doesn't know it, leaving him seemingly blameless if he "passes" it to another partner. Once again, women are dirty. Awesome.

It gets worse! You can also get a host of STIs from blow jobs or getting your clit licked. Yes, that's right. You're not safe during oral sex. Isn't that blessed? You may think you're being safe by using condoms during intercourse, but you can most definitely get an STI from oral sex as well. Chlamydia, HPV, herpes, trichomoniasis, and gonorrhea are all spread through skin-on-skin contact. HIV can be spread through semen if you have a cut or sore in your mouth.

I had a reader once ask me how to get one-night stands to go down on her. I wanted to give her some girl-power information, but the truth is that a guy you just met shouldn't go down on you (or you on him) for safety reasons. Unless you're going to use a female condom or barrier method . . . which we both know you're not going to do, bitch.

Are you going to forgo oral sex during casual hookups? No. Let's be real here.

I know you're probably not going to use a condom (male or female) during oral sex, but it's important to know that you're putting yourself at risk. It's better to have the facts, even if you're going to completely disregard them. I'd rather you know, wouldn't you?

I've always been pretty good about using condoms, but I'm not perfect. I mean, raise your hand if you've never had unprotected sex.

Yeah, that's what I thought. Sometimes you're impatient, can't find a rubber, or are too drunk to give a fuck. We have all been there.

All you can do is forgive *yourself*, get tested, then do what needs to be done to cure or treat the STI and move on with your life.

When I found out I had chlamydia, I was terrified to tell my partner. I worried that he would think I was a whore or blame me for being unsafe. But I had nothing to be ashamed of. We hadn't become exclusive until a few weeks before the test came back positive. I hadn't broken his trust. I hadn't cheated on him.

In fact, I had been relatively responsible. I went to my yearly ob-gyn appointment, I was tested, I informed him of the results, and I took the antibiotics needed to kill the bacteria. He was totally understanding, God bless him.

Having that conversation with the person you're dating is hard AF. It takes a lot of courage. There is so much stigma and shame associated with an STI. So here's a rundown of how to handle this tricky chat.

You need to have the conversation the minute you find out you have an STI. In a trusting, healthy relationship, honesty is key.

You don't have to ask for forgiveness. There is nothing to forgive. You just have to own up to your status, be honest AF, and take it from there. Trust me: There will be much worse things in this shitshow we call life.

How do you even bring it up? This is not exactly a sexy conversation to have. I get it.

Don't drag it out. Don't make a romantic dinner date just to tell your boyfriend you have HPV. Now is not the time for fumbling and avoidance. Just explain what the fuck is going on and hold your head high.

You need to have the conversation in person. This is not the time for a text message with a bunch of sad-face emojis. Ask your partner to hang out and do something low-key at your house. Start with the fact that you love and care about him or her. Keep calm and do not start crying (if you can help it).

This is a conversation, not your personal monologue. Let your partner contribute. Allow questions. This is an unusual milestone for both of you. Being able to take it together will ultimately bring you closer. It's not going to break you up as long as your partner actually gives a fuck about you and your relationship.

When I first told my boyfriend at the time that I had chlamydia, he had a lot of questions. He was in his twenties, but he still wasn't really sure what made this STI different from others, how you contracted it, and how it was subsequently treated.

The first thing I did was explain that my doctor had called in the antibiotics for both of us to take. He didn't need to be tested since he had been exposed already. The best course of action was for him to take a dose of the azithromycin. I gave him every fact he asked for, and when I didn't know an answer, I asked the internet.

When you're in a relationship, you're coming from a place of trust. You owe it to your partner to be honest and forthcoming with the information. Help your partner understand what you're going through; it will help you to make him or her understand. You're better together.

Something you should be sure to mention in your conversation with your partner is that if you've contracted an STI that can't be killed with a round of antibiotics, you should use protection to keep your partner safe. If you have genital herpes, don't have intercourse during an outbreak, and always use condoms. If you have HPV, use a condom to keep the other person HPV-free. Tell your partner you want to use condoms because you care about his or her safety and health.

If you don't tell your partner you have an STI, you are a piece of shit. For real. So don't do that.

You also *must* inform all of your sexual partners who may have been exposed. This sucks, and not enough people do it.

Accepting you have to do this is one thing; actually doing it is a whole other level of anxiety-inducing mayhem. Call them. Yes, on the actual phone. You don't send a text message in this situation for two reasons: First, it's fucking rude. You don't tell your partner you have an STI over text, and you don't tell someone you may have infected that you have an STI over a text. It's a health issue, and this person deserves to hear it out of your mouth, regardless of how meaningless the hookup may have been. Secondly, you do not want this person saving your message, text, or voice mail and attempting to shame you with it. I know this sounds exceptionally fucked up, but the lengths of degradation people will go to never ceases to astound. If you call this person, you can say what's up quickly. It is terrifying in the short term, but the evidence is nonexistent. I won't try to tell you that being honest won't end in public shame. It just might. Weaken the odds by turning them in your favor.

If you're anything like me, that list of people to call is likely pretty extensive. You'll quickly grow numb to anger. Make a list of everyone and start by calling the people you think are least angry first. What if they start getting super mad? Hold the phone six inches from your face so you can't hear them and say, "Would you rather I didn't tell you so you would be walking around with a possible STI and not know it?" If the person you're trying to be fucking truthful with is being a fucking asshole, *hang up the phone*. Go into the call history, scroll down, and block that fucker's number. Bye forever, dickwad!

You are not a coward. You are a strong, fierce-ass, nasty woman, and you are not going to pussy out and neglect to inform someone of his or her compromised physical health. It will likely be one of the most awkward, horrendously awful phone calls of your entire life, but it is better than being a coward.

Just like telling past partners may not go well, it may also go poorly when you share the news with your sex partner. This may go *very* badly. However, there is also a good chance it will not. I wish I could say that every partner is going to be understanding about an STI. According to a 2016 study from ZavaMed, which surveyed 1,700 people in the UK and United States, 43 percent of people say that an STI would be cause for breakup. What do you do if your partner freaks the fuck out?

Give him or her some space. This could be an emotional reaction, and your partner may need some time to process the facts. Finding out the person you're dating has an STI is pretty traumatizing. That's just the cold truth.

If your partner breaks up with you over an STI, he or she isn't someone you want to be with. How can you be with someone who can't handle a case of gonorrhea? How could you trust someone who won't be with you because you were honest about having genital herpes? If they can't take the information, good riddance. This person was obviously not for you. Imagine what would happen if a family member died or if you got cancer. This person you're dating clearly wouldn't have the chops to handle it.

Likewise, if a partner is open with you about their status, if they are vulnerable and honest enough to share that they have an STI, approach it with empathy. If you decide you don't want to continue the relationship, that's your choice. But there are ways to prevent the spread of STIs, and if you care about this person, it feels pretty unfair to write them off for an infection. Above all, approach them with empathy. You deserve it, and so do they.

Rejection fucking sucks. It might be the worst part of a breakup. It makes you feel dirty, worthless, and unlovable. Your STI status being the main culprit for a breakup will likely make you feel shitty. There isn't any way around those feelings. Just remember that you aren't alone. A lot of people have been in this position; 28 percent of people in the world currently have an incurable STI. We just don't talk about it enough, and that's why there is so much stigma. But there doesn't need to be.

For example, I was at a birthday party at a very fancy New York restaurant. The birthday girl was one of the coolest and most bad-ass women I know. She emanates fierceness and wears her vulner-abilities on her sleeve in a way I admire. Hers is the nasty-woman confidence I try to emulate every day.

Between sips of champagne and with bracelets jangling from her dainty wrist, she said, "Well, all the women in my family have herpes. It's a family thing. When my sister showed symptoms, she was freaking out. She was running cold water on her vagina in the bathtub, and my mother said, 'Welcome to the club, babe. All the Smith girls have herpes.'"

She said it so casually, like it was the simplest thing in the entire world. Meanwhile, I nearly spit my drink out of my nose. I didn't comment. She was so cool about it. What could I say to her? How could someone so glamorous have herpes?

I admired that she didn't let it bring her down. She didn't let it bring her family down. She still sparkled like a thousand suns under her thousand dollars' worth of jewelry. It didn't dim her shine because she didn't let it.

If you have an STI, you can live with it. Babe, you can *live* with HIV now. You don't have to wear your STI status as a badge of shame. Life is too short to let a condomless sex mistake ruin it.

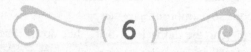

(6)

Masturbate Me Straight to Paradise

We aren't being political enough about female masturbation and orgasm. Sexual positivity isn't built upon what it needs to be on. I really believe about sexual empowerment as starting with real, real self-love. Not just about, "I can have an orgasm because I'm really turned on," but "I'm in love with my body, I love myself, I love how I feel, I know what makes me feel good."
—Claire Cavanah, cofounder of Babeland

I remember the first time I discovered my clitoris. I was six years old. I climbed onto one of the oak posters of my parents' four-poster bed, probably pretending to be a Disney villain. (I always identified more with Maleficent and Ursula. I don't know why my child psychologist was surprised by this; my mother only wore gothic couture when I was growing up.)

As I ascended the pole, legs wrapped around, I realized it felt really amazing, electrifying, even. It was different from anything I'd ever experienced. It was ecstasy. Better than ice cream, better than candy, better than anything in the whole world.

Though I've grown into my adult life and my parents are very open about sex, no one bothered to inform me when I was a little girl that what I was experiencing was an orgasm: a perfectly normal and delightful part of human existence. I had to figure it all out on my own through masturbation and outside research. I have parents who talk about sex, and I still didn't know jack shit. This is partially why I became a sex educator and writer. We're seriously missing some shit in our sex education, and it's harming us in ways we have trouble grasping.

In all of our (profoundly little and profoundly lacking) sex education, we never teach young people about pleasure. We don't bother to tell them about their hot spots because we're far too busy telling them not to touch them . . . or each other's. We're focused on keeping them STI- and pregnancy-free. While this is important, it doesn't make teaching about things beyond this curriculum any less critical.

We have got to stop focusing on penetration so aggressively and get back to the basics. Penetrative sex doesn't deliver female orgasms the vast majority of the time. I know we're a little old for sex education, but a refresher isn't going to hurt you. Plus, you're reading this book like, now. You know what's up. You'll likely learn something. If there is one thing I've figured out through teaching about and writing about sex, it's that there is always something new to discover. Let's party.

On the next page is a diagram of genital anatomy for people who own vulvas.

When you have penetrative sex, the penis goes into the vaginal opening. You can see it there, right? Now, locate the clitoris. Do you see how fucking high up the clitoris is from the vagina in the picture?

Two in three people with vulvas require clitoral stimulation in order to orgasm. Pleasure is what the clit was designed for. It's literally its only function. You can't (usually) reach the clitoris through

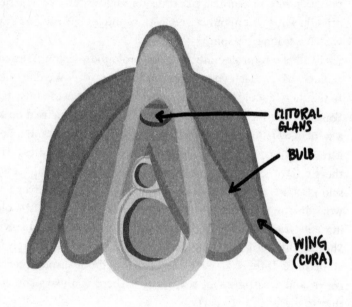

a straight-up dicking. It's really just not physically possible, unless you're actually taking the clitoris into account when choosing sex positions or bringing a vibrator into the bedroom to make up the difference. Imagine how much better sex would have been when we were younger if only we'd been taught what a clit is, am I right?!

When we spend so much time teaching about straight-up hetero sex (vaginal intercourse), we're not teaching women how to have orgasms. If you're only teaching girls and boys how to have sex in a manner that's entirely focused on a boy's pleasure, what is that telling young women about their own orgasms?

It's indirectly teaching them they aren't as important. Fuck that. You can bet this lack of emphasis affects a woman's confidence. If a woman is taught that her pleasure comes secondary to a man's, it reinforces male-centric ideas that her orgasm is not critical to the sexual process. She begins to think of herself (however subconsciously) as less worthy than her male counterparts. This makes a woman an object; it makes her a means to an end, with that end being the male orgasm. And that could not be further from the truth. She is a majestic queen and should be coming every single time.

A confident woman is fostered by positive reinforcement. Her confidence is made strong by the people and educators around her that are telling her it is okay to put herself first, to seek satisfaction and think of herself as the primary vessel of her own pleasure. She is not supposed to just lie there while some sweaty dude humps her like a jackhammer.

We need to instill these values to fortify the strength all women have but are rarely encouraged to explore and grasp onto. By teaching a woman about herself and her value, we resolve to rebuild her confidence. And, you know, high-key topple the Patriarchy like we talked about in chapters 1 and 2.

We've got to reevaluate what we're teaching young people. Girls need to be taught what a clitoris is right off the bat. Masturbation is a building block of self-esteem. It teaches young women that they don't need a boy in order to feel pleasure, that they can give it to themselves. That's a really profound and amazing message to teach young women. In a time when women are marginalized and controlled by their sexuality, giving them the tools they need to make themselves happy is fucking crucial.

Our society doesn't teach this to young girls because it would give them free range over their own bodies. In a world that constantly seeks to control and manipulate how we interact with and perceive our bodies, giving women the tools they need for self-satisfaction is dangerous. What will the little boys do if girls figure out they can come like crazy by pressing just one button?

Once you learn where your clitoris and G-spot are located and how they work, it's time to actually use them. It's time to bring masturbation out of the Dark Ages and into the glorious, vibrator-abundant world.

MASTURBATION IS HOT FOR ONE AND ALL

Ladies, you've got to masturbate regularly. This is one of the first steps toward reclaiming your identity and understanding your body. When used to enhance your knowledge of what makes your body tick, masturbation will only make your sex life better. It helps you communicate because you know what you want. If you don't know what you like and don't know how you like to be touched, how the fuck can you tell another person what you like?

Every single vagina is different. Different women want and enjoy different things. You have to spend time with yourself and actually discover those pleasure points in order to own them. There is nothing sexier than a woman who knows her own body. If you're with a partner who doesn't feel that your sexual literacy is hot, don't date that person. He or she is being a fucking idiot.

And if you really need to convince someone why masturbation is important and fabulous and amazing, you can always cite the health benefits.

The way to make sex culturally acceptable is to focus on the provable benefits erotic pleasure has on the mind and body. Health, people! Your soul will not be damned, but your cardiovascular health will be improved greatly!

Orgasms are one of life's natural pleasures; they are part of the beautiful existence of humanity. According to a 2009 study published in the *Journal of Sexual Medicine,* orgasms were shown to increase the flow of neurotransmitters and flood the brain with feel-good chemicals. Your brain releases oxytocin, a natural pain reliever and pair-bonding hormone, your anxiety reduces, and you chill out. Climax also releases endorphins and dopamine, which can greatly reduce stress. When you come, the world is just straight-up better.

Though there isn't irrefutable evidence to prove this, some experts say that masturbation can help women flush bacteria out of their cervix, which can improve overall vaginal health. When you are aroused, your cervix naturally opens slightly. This opening (called *tenting*) improves cervical circulation and can help push out bacteria that may be gathered. Pretty dope, right? The female body is amazing. I just had to say it (again).

Masturbation can also make your sex life with your partner better. According to a 2003 article published in the *Journal of Psychology and Human Sexuality,* self-love was found to increase sexual well-ness for couples. While the reasons for this are many, it has a lot to do with the idea that if you're having great sex, you want to masturbate (with and/or without your partner present). And if you're masturbating, you want to have more sex. While this isn't true of all couples, sex is often something you just want more of. And the more you're engaging with your body on a personal level, the more you'll want to fuck your partner.

And, babe, it all comes back to that "knowing yourself" thing we talked about earlier; if you know what you like after masturbating, you'll be interested in communicating those newfound plea-sure points with your partner. If you test out your sexual curiosities on yourself, you can bring them to your partner when you're ready to get down and nasty.

Self-love should be one of the first lessons mothers teach their daughters when they're entering puberty (but honestly, probably around six or seven). Awkward AF conversation? Maybe. But, like most things, it will become normal if you just do it.

We live in an age when we're finally being encouraged to en-gage in self-care. From brunch with the girls to lighting aromather-apy candles, to writing in a journal, to having a cathartic emotional cry, women across the country are taking a minute for themselves. Trust me, you won't miss the hashtags on Instagram if you're look-ing for them. Self-care is the new pumpkin spice latte—the staple for basic bitches everywhere.

Basicness aside, this is fucking awesome. I'm so happy to see women focusing on themselves for once and actually putting their own needs and desires above those around them. But why isn't masturbation included among those sacred rituals?

If we allow orgasms to carry their full weight—if we stop trivializing their importance and actually start making them a part of every single #SelfCareSunday—they will start having a positive impact on our health, minds, and bodies. Masturbation shouldn't be something you're only doing in the dead of night, to girl-on-girl porno on RedTube, with headphones strapped in and hiding like some kind of dirty creep (unless you're into that exact scenario—or have roommates. Honestly, however whacking off turns you on or is convenient is great). You should be able to put masturbation on a fucking to-do list.

Manicure? Check. Shopping for that new sweater? Check. Gym? Check. Coming my face off? *Check.*

Sounds pretty great to me. Self-love is your biologically ingrained meditation. Don't deny yourself the opportunity. Discover what you like, take time for yourself, and really let your mind engage in a dialogue with your body. There is nothing to be ashamed of; you're (literally) just doing you.

Since you're doing you . . . you should have the tools that suit *you*. This is a purchase that is for you and no one else. Go forth and make it worthwhile.

Now, we live in a time that isn't making us horny right now. I get that. I have to concentrate on masturbation and schedule it into my life sometimes. In 2017, women's sexual health and wellness company Unbound did a survey of over five hundred women to figure out how the election of El Presidente Cheeto was affecting female libido. In the survey, 27 percent said they masturbated less, and 18 percent said their enjoyment of sexual activity had decreased. We cannot let this fuckface get us to turn away from our pussies. No. They don't deserve that, you guys.

We all need to buy new vibrators, reclaim our sexuality, and show this fucker what we're made of—orgasms and stardust.

GET THE RIGHT VIBE AND
FALL IN LOVE WITH IT

According to a survey from the Center for Sexual Health Promotion at Indiana University in Bloomington, 47 percent of women still don't own a vibrator. A separate survey conducted by Adam and Eve found that nearly 56 percent of women don't own a vibrator. That is, in a word, fucked. Both of those figures are bleak. So what the hell?

The thing that deters a lot of women from proper masturbation is the actual purchasing of a vibrator. It's such a cause for concern for so many of us. No one wants to be seen buying something they're going to use to get themselves off. Yes, your fingers are magical things as well, but if you're denying yourself a (wo)man-made tool because you're *afraid,* then no, honey. Just no.

We've got to remove the stigma. We should be talking about our vibrators like we talk about a new pair of shoes. I make it a point to tell women what I'm buying, the new things I'm trying, and what they should be purchasing for their goodie drawers. If we talk about it, it stops being icky.

Finding the right vibrator is like finding the right life partner. It brings you to new heights, inspires you, and shows you what you're really capable of. It's fucking liberating as hell, and we all deserve liberation and pussy agency.

The relationship you have with your vibrator is as important as the relationship you have with the lady who does your eyebrows: trusted, necessary, and always there for you in your hairiest moments. (Don't get me started on the patriarchal backdrop that serves as the foundation for our pathological need for hair grooming or we'll never get to vibrators.)

A vibe is the core tool that brings you closer to self-love. It's the thing that makes breaking up with that fuckboy stop feeling like the end of the world. If you have an orgasm at home, what's to keep you in a shitty dating situation?

You need to find a vibe you can trust—one you can spend a whole afternoon with and not ever want to be apart from.

So don't take the purchasing process lightly.

Go out and buy yourself a nice-ass piece of equipment. You don't have to be a seedy piece of shit when you're buying a vibrator. You don't have to go to one of those garbage places with the sex doll in the window that's wearing a sexy cop uniform. You don't have to walk into a sketchy corner shop with a full-case plexiglass display of bongs and giant black dildos to get a proper vibe. We've moved on from that. Sex isn't gross. Sex is life.

There are real, legitimate boutiques for this shit now. Go on Google and search for a local sex-toy boutique. Now, not every place has them. If you're not in a major city, you might have difficulty finding a spot to shop. If this is the case, welcome to the internet. Get on lewandmassager.com and get yourself a wand massager. This vibrator will never let you down.

For a beginner, get something nonthreatening. The Magic Wand, Le Wand, or any wand toy looks like a neck massager, but it's pretty fucking sizable. For some women, it's a scary thought to put that thing near your clitoris. The first time I went to use a Hitachi, I thought I might burn off my clitoris. FYI: This is not the thought you're supposed to have when you're getting ready to masturbate.

If you want something unassuming, get yourself a bullet vibe. Bullet vibes are small, portable, and come in adorable, nonthreatening colors (like hot pink and aquamarine). Some of them even have little bunny ears that go on either side of your clit. It looks like a little rabbit; what could be terrifying about that? I have one that looks like an actual lipstick. I can carry it around in my purse, and no one has any idea it's a sex toy.

A thing to understand is that a vibrator is an *investment*. You'll definitely be able to find some vibes that are cheap, require batteries instead of a USB connector, and are made with fewer high-quality materials. But don't buy that trash.

Choose a vibrator that is made from medical-grade silicone, uses an actual charge to reboot, and has different speeds and range of motion (if you're going for something a little more advanced). You do *not* have to buy one that looks like a porn star's dick, okay? This should be fun, not traumatizing.

When it comes to your self-care, you take it seriously, right? You invest in it. The same should be true for masturbation. Give a girl the right vibrator, and she can rule the world.

You'll end up saving money in the long run because you won't be up shit creek without an orgasm and having to replace your shitty discount vibe because you didn't want to invest in your vagina/vulva. Invest in yourself, girl!

LEARN ABOUT YOUR BODY
AND REALLY LISTEN TO IT

The clitoris is a glorious, beautiful iceberg: solitary and complicated. That little, magical, rosebud-like, crown-jewel-esque bead atop the labia minora is just the tip of a rather large pleasure center.

On the next page is a diagram of the clitoris.

As you can see, only the glans clitoris is visible on the outside of the body. The wings on either side are hidden within. What so many people don't know is that the visible part of the majestic AF clit is not all there is to it. You know how you find the rest of it? By exploring your anatomy. It's up to five inches in some women! That's legit the size of an average peen. Take a hand mirror and look at your vulva. Get to know what it looks like and accept it. Every vulva is different, and every single one is beautiful. Next, touch yourself. Try different things. Touch different areas of the vulva and pay attention to the way your body responds. Start with the clitoris. Begin with a light circular motion over the glans and see how that feels. Don't be afraid to explore whatever feels good. You can also touch the labia, the vaginal opening, or insert one or two fingers into the vagina.

This means getting down with your bad self and actually spending some time masturbating. You should be "allowing" for masturbation or even scheduling it between hot yoga and scrolling through your Twitter feed. It should be a natural part of your routine. It should be something you go to as a pastime, like catching up on your favorite Netflix drama.

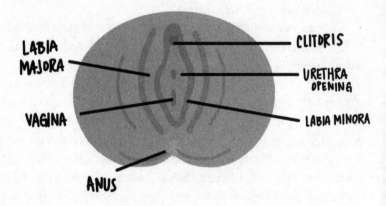

HOW TO MAKE IT SEXIER THAN A SEX SCENE ON TRENCHCOATX

There are so many fabulous ways to get yourself off. It goes so beyond lying in the lotus position, legs spread, fantasizing about some sexy actor, and figuring out what works for you.

You don't just have that little bud on top. Go deeper than that. Move the vibrator down into different areas of the labia. See what feels good for you. Your pussy is as unique as a snowflake, so find out what turns it into a shooting star. If you can't send yourself to outer space, you think some guy or girl is going to pull it off? Hell no.

Here are a few of my favorite techniques I learned from Alex Fine, cofounder of Dame Products and consummate badass bitch (you can also find these techniques at OMGYES.com):

Grounding: Instead of going full clit, take three fingers or your palm (whichever you prefer) and press into your vagina. A deeper, more grounded feel may be more pleasurable for you. Direct stimulation can be overwhelming.

Orbiting: Don't directly touch the clitoris at all if it feels like too much. Instead, orbit the clitoris in a figure eight. It builds the pleasure up but doesn't overstimulate a sensitive clit.

Tapping: Maybe you don't like rubbing at all. That's cool. You don't have to rub your clit. You can also gently tap it;

giving it a brief sensation and then taking it away. You can build to orgasm this way.

Layering: Take the labia majora and/or labia minora and layer it over the clit. This may take some tinkering to find what really works for you. Don't be shy! It's just your vulva, remember? Having an extra barrier between your fingers and toys to the clitoris is a better way to achieve orgasm for many women.

You don't just have to lie there on your back with your legs butterflied. You can jazz up your self-sex, too. Try different positions. Instead of being on your back, try all fours. Reach through your legs and pleasure yourself this way. Try leaning your vibrator against a chair and grinding against it, or go all the way and fuck it.

One of the scariest and most beautiful things about female anatomy is that the possibilities are truly endless. The key is to just try a bunch of different shit and see what works. Not everything will work; some things will feel really weird and uncomfortable. That is totally okay. You won't know until you try. When it comes to self-love, the last thing you should be is intimidated. It's your body, and you have got to know what makes it tick.

I'm going to drop the P-word now—are you ready? *Porn.* Fantasies you create in your mind are fucking stellar, but porn is the shit. I know a lot of you sexy, badass ladies shy away from porn or don't want to talk about what you're watching.

Ladies, there is nothing wrong with masturbation, and there is nothing wrong with porn. Sure, there is plenty of shit out there that is straight-up gross. As feminist entrepreneur and sex genius Cindy Gallop has said to me in the approximately fifty times I've interviewed her, the terrible, piece-of-crap porn movies we see are not inherently a porn problem but a porn *industry* problem.

These corporate dudes think that men want a certain kind of movie and then mass-produce that same, bad-quality bullshit over and over again. They think every single man wants to see a scene wherein two guys double-team an unrealistically large-breasted blond woman. Consent is seemingly optional in many of these scenes. One time I was watching a video on one of those shitty free sites (Pornhub, maybe), where this teenager started having sex with her friend's dad. While growing up I thought something like that was super hot in 90s movies like *Poison Ivy* with Drew Barrymore, but looking at this scene as an adult was kind of . . . gross. I know we all have fantasies and I'm all about opening yourself up to all sorts of mental images, but fucking a fourteen-year-old and genuinely thinking that written script was hot enough to make a movie is gnarly. Hard pass.

It's not even necessarily men who want this as their erotic material. Frankly, no one gives a shit as long as they make money. This crap is what corporations think men want to see. I love a good porn video, and I still know this is sick and gross.

Luckily, there are other options. Indie porn, if you will. Pioneers like Erika Lust, TRENCHCOATx, and many more are making female-focused, queer-friendly porn that is high quality and straight-up hot. Just the other day, I watched a scene on TRENCH-COATx where the couple not only had damn near panty-soaking sex but there was cunnilingus and true-to-life passion. It's such a game changer. Porn that is made ethically is important. We need to make more of an effort to watch things that are good for us—things that actually turn *us* on. The clitoris is front and center! It's magical.

Porn can be used in a healthy way, and it can really amp up your self-love experiences. Porn is the same as many outside substances—it enhances the experience as long as it is used in moderation and isn't interfering with your life. If you enjoy porn, that's super awesome. We all have a freak flag; we're just afraid to fly it. Ask your friends for recommendations. Look at porn made for women (yes, this is a thing). Erika Lust is my all-time girl crush. She is a feminist pornographer, and her stuff is . . . um, I'll be right back.

Porn only becomes a problem if it's negatively affecting your real sex life and harming your relationship with your partner. Porn can be superhot; you just have to be aware of how you're using it. There are certainly ways in which porn can become harmful. Sex addiction is a real thing, but it's pretty rare. It's more of a compulsive behavior. Pay attention to how often you're watching porn. As long as you use it as a form of entertainment and don't let it overtake your entire life and allow your real sex life to suffer, you're all right. Society loves to shame people who watch porn and to call them sexual deviants. This just isn't true. Porn is a fantasy. It is entertainment just like any other movie. You watch *Kill Bill* for the violence and kick-ass fight scenes; you watch porn for the intense, hard-core sex scenes.

Almost all porn is made for consumption by men, so finding something you like can be intimidating. There are only so many violent gang bangs you can fast-forward through before you're ready to call it quits (unless you're into violent gang bangs, which is totally fine, too).

Being willing to slough through all the shitty, bad acting and female degradation (I get full-body shivers when I think about this one fisting video I came upon by chance) is half the battle. If you keep an open mind and scroll through RedTube for a while, eventually you'll happen upon something you like. There is some good stuff out there, I promise. It just takes digging.

To be honest, half the sick and twisted stuff you see in porn is actually pretty lady-boner inducing if you give it a chance. I'm not saying you may necessarily be turned on by a scripted scene wherein a woman does not want a guy anally penetrating her like the example above, but it is just a movie. You don't have to feel badly about the defilement of your fellow female; she's a professional porn actress. We all revel in the taboo and seedy. It's okay, bb.

If you can't deal with the crappy quality, amateur shitstorm that is free porn, get a subscription. Lord knows, it's the ads on RedTube that get me the hottest. I love me some HD peen.

If you complain about how terrible porn is but aren't willing to pay for the good stuff, you're making a shitty argument, and I don't feel bad for you. It's impossible to take your ass seriously, girl. Good porn is not even expensive. Check out EroticaX, Kink, and other high-quality sites. It's worth it. I love them. I use them more than my Netflix account, and it's marginally more pricey.

MAKE MASTURBATION PART OF YOUR CONVERSATION

The other day, I was having dinner with one of my old friends from my internship days back in college. We were enjoying our red and green curry in a cheap Thai restaurant near NYU. I brought up masturbation, as I always tend to do. As I regaled her with stories of my latest and greatest discoveries on the vibrator market, she began looking pretty distraught.

Did I stop talking about it? No. I called her out for being awkward. I changed the entire dynamic. What, I can't talk about my pussy in a restaurant in New York City? I refuse to adhere to such a stupid standard. Perhaps masturbation isn't a complementary aperitif to Thai cuisine, but if being extreme is what it takes to get other women to acknowledge their sex organs, I'm going to fucking do it.

Start talking about it! And don't stop fucking talking about it! Make masturbation a part of your everyday conversation.

You don't have to discuss pussy power over cocktails every time you meet up with a friend, but you shouldn't be afraid to talk about it. Once we add these ideas into our everyday cultural lexicon, we'll finally be able to think about masturbation and pleasure without shame. It's only when the ideas stop being disgraceful that they can stop being scary. That is the world I want to live in. It's the world we sexually empowered women deserve. How else can we really thrive?

It will take a lot of work and time to make female sexuality just another important part of our everyday list of conversational topics, but the more we discuss it, the closer we get. Make people a little uncomfortable. If they can't handle the heat, it's probably because they haven't been orgasming enough.

Pussy power. It's the only way to live.

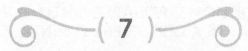

Nasty Women Don't Skimp on the Stuff That Makes Sex Better

Calling all females! It's me, Gigi. Here with a bedazzled microphone ready to tell you that you need more *moisture* in your life. Do you own lube? And I don't mean a little lube. I mean a *lot* of lube. Lube in big bottles, in medium-size bottles, lube in travel sizes. Lube is everything, the elixir of life, the barrier against clit friction, the sauce that keeps the vaginal tissues from tearing.

Lube me up before you do anything to my body. I ain't trying to get no road rash up on my coochie, ya hear? Condoms are not optional. Lube is not optional. When the actual fuck did everyone stop using condoms? Why doesn't anyone know about lube? This is an act of domestic terror against our pussies, my friends!

We've talked about masturbation and pleasure; we're going to get into kink later. All of these things should be coated in a heavy layer of lube. Even sexting should be metaphorically lubed up.

YO, CONDOMS! RELIABLE BIRTH CONTROL IS A GIRL'S BEST FRIEND

But about condoms and reliable birth control real quick. You'll see how all of these things connect, I promise.

I'm sitting in an ice cream parlor with one of my friends, at her birthday dinner, when she revealed she uses the pull-and-pray method. She was pretty lit in her skintight Baby Spice party dress. We were seated, a giant group of girls, in a sugar-themed restaurant. What was a lovely evening turned into my leading a charge of five girls explaining how stupid this was and why she needed to get her shit together. Sorry not sorry. I'm a sex educator and sexologist, and I can't have one of my idiot friends thinking this is fine. Bad timing? Yeah, probably. Still don't care. Meanwhile, her confused and petrified boyfriend sat by, as pale as the unused condoms in his bedside drawer.

A few weeks later, I'm scrolling through Instagram and coming across an ad for some app called something like Natural Woman or Organic Pussy or something equally lame. The ad claimed that it could tell you if you were fertile by taking your temperature. It claimed to be the "only certified app" for your cycle and promised it was a great natural alternative to other birth control. Certified by what? The Dumbass Society, USA? It was created by a doctor, so while I'm sure there is some merit to this idea, it's not a good idea. It's just not. Does your temperature rise during ovulation? Yes. Do sperm live inside your body for up to five days after ejaculation and therefore could be in there waiting to pounce post-ovulation? Yes.

But, Gigi, you're not a doctor! Neither are you, honey.

There is a whole movement right now about measuring your natural cycles and going on the rhythm method. Stupid. Not a good idea. I'm not saying it's impossible to use this method, but that doesn't make it healthy or a reliable form of birth control. I have to hand it to women who can track their cycles and it works for them. This takes excellent skills in managing your cycle's schedule, really, REALLY fucking knowing exactly when your period comes every single month, and REMEMBERING to update your apps and calendars. Most women can't remember to take a goddamn pill at the same time every day, let alone track a cycle.

Taking your temperature to see if you're fertile? Are you fucking kidding me? Do you have any idea how many unplanned pregnancies would result because of this absurd, irresponsible iPhone application? Yes, your body goes through cycles wherein you're more fertile than other times, but this does not mean you cannot conceive. It may be much less likely, but it's still possible. Even though pills, patches, IUDs, implants, and condoms were all funded by male-owned companies and created by people without vaginas, it doesn't mean you get to just skip out on birth control and call it a day. You need a reliable form of birth control. You need to take your body and physical health into your own hands. Are you seriously going to trust someone with your safety like that?

As one of my old friends from high school told me on Facebook when I wrote about the pull-out method some years ago, "That is how I got my mini me." As in, how she got her kid.

On top of being fed ridiculous shit like the aforementioned, people don't even know how to use many forms of birth control properly. Data from the University of Indiana, wherein researchers studied fifty different outside studies on condom usage, found that more than 57 percent of people put condoms on wrong (and I am being conservative here. Other researchers and medical professionals put the error margin more toward 75–85 percent). If that many people are fucking up condoms, do you really think people are going to be able to handle the rhythm method? Sperm lives inside you for three to five days. Are you really going to take the risk of being off by one or two days? Is that something you want to be responsible for? Doctors I've spoken to have told me that having a form of birth control you trust can make sex better because it takes away the constant, burdening fear of getting pregnant. Personally, I'd have an anxiety attack every single time someone got near me with a penis if I weren't strapped with my birth control pills. No thanks. Not into it. That's canceled.

Which brings me back to my earlier, possibly alienating (hey, I'll take it) statement, which I've now rephrased as a question: Yo, ladies! When the actual fuck did everyone stop using condoms? What, condoms went out of style in 2006 like JNCO jeans and low-rise leather pants? PSA: Condoms are *not* optional. Birth control is *not* optional. Lube is *not* optional.

CONDOMS AND WHY YOU NEED THEM

Condoms are not bikini waxes. They are not something you get to decide to use sometimes and other times, you just go free. They are not an "if I feel like it" kind of a thing. They are a must. The saddest part is that we've made condoms so unsexy that no one wants to use them.

It's fucked up that we live in a sex-negative culture where people think condoms are not a big deal, that they make sex bad, that they don't protect from STIs anyway (my personal fav), and are now just another thing men manipulate their way out of.

Education is obviously doing essentially nothing to help on this one. Neurotic parents and religious leaders would rather tell people nothing at all about safe sex than mention condoms. *No sex until you're married or you'll go to hell, Maria! The Pill will make you infertile or give you cancer, Darlene!*

Condoms are a huge fucking deal. News flash: People are going to fuck each other whether or not they know how to do it safely. Humans are sexual beings. This is a universal truth of life. People like to fuck. They are never going to not fuck. This is an empirical fact that has been so since the dawn of the humanoids who lived in trees. Honestly, if we stop pretending that all people don't love sex and that people are going to do it, we'd be so much better off. Your clit offers a high that is free, healthy, and always available. Don't even tell me people aren't into getting off. Don't try me.

Instead of thinking that condoms are a nonmandatory form of birth control and STI protection, do yourself a favor and stop being a fucking idiot.

1-800-SHUT-THE ext. FUCKUP. It doesn't matter which birth control you use (but you should use one), but condoms are the only way you're going to prevent STDs and STIs. Condoms are 98 percent effective at preventing pregnancy and (most—we'll get to that) STIs when used correctly. Do you know how well the Pill prevents STIs? Zero percent. Any guesses on how well an IUD prevents STIs? Literally 0 percent effective. Want to wager a bet on how well the pull-out method works to prevent infections? Works 0 percent.

BULLSHIT EXCUSES PEOPLE USE FOR NOT USING CONDOMS AND WHY THEY ARE, IN FACT, A LOAD OF BULLSHIT

Condoms don't feel good on. It makes sex feel like nothing on my dick. :(

Bullshit. Hm. Is that so? Why is it that penis-owning people can have orgasms while wearing condoms if this is the case? If wearing a condom makes sex so terrible, why do you still come? I call bullshit on this bullshit. Condoms do not make sex worse. They don't. This is a myth. I know, I know. I don't own a penis, so how can I know? Please see above.

Now, I'd be lying if I said condoms didn't dry things out and add a barrier between penis and vulva/vagina. They do that. It's true. Obviously, barebacking is the "natural" state, and if the world weren't a festering colony of viruses and bacteria, we could all just do whatever. But it is, and we can't. Dryness and constriction aside, it doesn't mean we don't need to use them. Get an ultrathin condom. Read everything I have to say about lube on the following pages. You need lube even when you don't use condoms with a long-term partner. Don't be dumb. Don't. Be. Dumb. Dontbedumb.

But, he says he was tested just a few weeks ago and I totally trust him! He's just not that kind of person. Trust me. I know him. You don't understand.

Bullshit. You've been dating a millisecond. What are you even fucking talking about?

Do not trust anyone who tells you they have been tested. I know I've mentioned this before, but it cannot be said enough. Unless someone shows you a clean bill of health (I'm talking medical records) and is having sex exclusively with you, condoms are not up for negotiation. How could he possibly know that he's clean? As I've mentioned before and will (probably) mention again and again until I die, men can't even be tested for HPV. That's right. A man can have HPV and not even be aware. Pass.

We just had a whole talk about STDs and STIs. You read a whole goddamn chapter about this. Do you want an STI? Seriously. No, seriously, I'm asking.

I'm allergic to latex.

Bullshit. According to the American Latex Allergy Association, 1 percent of the entire population has a latex allergy. Bye, Felicia. There are condoms made of polyurethane, too. Latex-free, bitch. It's just as effective, but not made of latex. Again, bye. *Bye.*

Don't you trust me?

Bullshit. Also, fuck you. Guilting someone into going bareback with you is a pretty shitty thing to do. It doesn't matter how much you think you trust someone, you need to use condoms. It is completely possible that this person really does think he or she is clean. STIs don't always show symptoms. As I already covered in chapter 5, many don't. Your health is too precious of a thing to risk. Bottom line.

Carry condoms in your wallet. There are even feminist condoms now. Lovability makes condoms that say empowering shit like, "No fuckboys allowed!" A woman who carries condoms has long been stigmatized. You're a "loose woman" if you're prepared for life. Why would a suitable wife and mother be carrying around condoms? You must be easy and down for anything if you carry condoms, right? Fuck that. You might be DTF (down to fuck), but you care about your sexual health and aren't about to let some fuckwad you just met give you something that doesn't come with a gift receipt.

Follow the directions for storage. Keep your purse condoms out of the sun when possible. Have a bowl of condoms at home on your nightstand like it's a housing décor choice. Make it part of the aesthetic. Condom chic.

Put a condom on your partner yourself. Learn how to put one by. There are plenty of YouTube videos devoted to condoms. Be sure to pinch the tip of the condom and roll it down over the full shaft of the penis.

Wear a condom the whole time during sex. A study published by the Society of Family Planning found that only 59 percent of people wear condoms for the entire duration of intercourse. That has about zero chill.

Additionally, there is an incredibly fucked-up phenomenon call *stealthing*, wherein a partner takes a condom off without telling the person they're having sex with. Make no mistake—this is sexual assault. Anyone who removes a condom without your knowledge or says they've put a condom on when they really haven't is a disgusting piece of shit and deserves to be flown to Asshole Island and left there to fester and die.

SO, LUBE! . . . AND HOW CONDOMS AND LUBE GO TOGETHER LIKE CLITORISES AND VIBRATORS

Lube me up before you go, go. Lube me, baby, one more time. I should have been a poet. Oh, wait, those aren't my lines, are they? Lube, guys. Lube should go inside and outside of the condom.

Even lubricated condoms will dry your pussy out faster than a touch-up at Drybar. The gross lube that is on most condoms contains petrochemicals, glycerin, and parabens. None of these things are good for the temperamental vaginal ecosystem (more on that later). But worse still? Condoms without lube can get dry (or even drier) and then tear.

Don't just lube up the outside; lube up the inside to make it feel better for both of you. Stay away from silicone-based lubes or coconut oil. Most silicone lubes are condom-safe, but some have a higher oil content than others, which can fuck you up. Oil corrodes latex and causes condoms to break. The more you know.

Don't forget to check the expiration date. This is a mistake many people make. If your condom is past the expiration date, it is more likely to break. Most packs of condoms are less than ten dollars. It's not going to break the bank to buy new ones.

As I said about the purse thing, always store your condoms in a cool, dry place. Carrying them around in your purse for extended periods of time, only to whip them out at a music festival à la *Bridget Jones's Baby*, is less than ideal. You don't need to be hypomanic about the condoms' expiration date, just keep it in mind and always be aware. Condoms have a shelf life of five years. You're not that likely to have the same condoms for that long, anyway.

Take the time to find condoms that work for you. So many of these shitty brands make terrible condoms that screw with your pH balance and make sex awful. What you might not be aware of is that there are hundreds of different condoms to choose from (that might be an exaggeration, but it probably isn't). There is always a brand that will work for your specific needs. You don't have to buy Trojans just because an advertisement told you to nine hundred times. I keep thinking about the Trojan character from my youth singing, "Trojan Man!" and it makes me want to die. Trojans weren't designed for women. Case in point: Her Pleasure condoms with the "intensifying" lube that makes your pussy feel like it's been lit on fire with gasoline.

In a perfect world, we'd have something better than condoms. Condoms don't cover the balls or taint and can't protect 100 percent from the herpes virus. They also aren't perfect for preventing HPV, as HPV can be transmitted through skin-on-skin contact (be sure you got your HPV vaccinations, even though you're probably screwed on this one regardless). They aren't perfect. Maybe one day we'll have something better than condoms, but that day is not today.

Yeah, maybe one day the great scientists of the world will create immunizations for every STI known to (wo)man. In a perfect world, yes. I want that. I really do.

If you are having sex and exploring your sexual freedom, you need to be using condoms. I don't know when condoms stopped being something people thought they needed, but you need condoms. We need to make condoms sexy again. Sexual health is hot. Protecting and respecting your partner should be a turn-on.

Don't be a stupid bitch. And don't believe any idiot who says he needs Magnums. According to a study conducted in 2015 by Millward Brown, 25 percent of men in the United States have tried Magnum condoms. Meanwhile, the average dick size is 5.5 inches. Something isn't right here. There is nothing wrong with using regular condoms. If we didn't put so much pressure on men and all penis owners to have gigantic penises, they wouldn't feel the need to buy Magnums and risk having slippage. When we put unwarranted pressures on either sex, we all wind up fucked over. I don't have stats on this, but I'm guessing about 0.8 out of every 200 guys who says he needs Magnums actually does.

LET'S TALK MORE ABOUT LUBE.
LET'S BE LUBE EXPERTS!

I once had a guy tell me lube was insulting because he was sure he could make me wet enough. I'm still shaking my head. Lube is a threat to masculinity now?

'Tis, it seems. The story above is directly responsible for what happened a few years later. I was hooking up with this guy on Halloween weekend up in Milwaukee, Wisconsin, where I was visiting a friend at Marquette University. We'd been casually flirting for the last few nights and drunkenly making out. On the third night, I went home with him. We were having sex, and try as I might, I just couldn't get wet. Alcohol, cigarettes, and nerves do not make for a wet puss. I was so self-conscious. I didn't know how to ask to use lube. I didn't know that I even could ask to use lube or that I could say the sex was painful.

I'm sure he realized what was going on, but neither one of us said anything. He kept asking if I was okay and if it was "good" for me. I said it was because I didn't know what else to say. He just kept humping away, and I pretended like I wasn't counting the seconds until it was over. Neither he nor I had the language or emotional intelligence to communicate what was happening, which would have allowed us to remedy the situation. We just kept going at it like a couple of idiots.

I don't know about him (and obviously give not one single F about that rando), but I was embarrassed, and it made the encounter damaging both physically and emotionally. I didn't end up seeing him again for a myriad of reasons, but the main reason was because I now associated him with shame, discomfort, and awkwardness. No sexual experience should make you feel badly or ashamed of yourself. Even now, I look back on that night nearly ten years ago and I cringe.

So from this story, I genuinely hope you will walk away with a newfound appreciation for lube. Lube is the unsung hero of sex. She deserves all the snaps.

WHY LUBE IS SO IMPORTANT

Not everyone will experience a sandpaper sexcape like the one I described above, but that doesn't mean you shouldn't invite lube into your sex life. When aroused, blood rushes to the genitals and causes them to swell and lubricate for intercourse. Your vagina naturally lubricates, which is great, but it rarely lubricates enough, yet another contributing factor to scarce female orgasms during intercourse. When it comes to sex, wetter is better. Lube takes away all the guesswork and pressure to turn someone on "enough." Sometimes our brains don't match up to our bodies. Maybe your boyfriend or girlfriend just spent twenty minutes with his or her head between your legs and you're still not wet. It happens. It happens to me all the time. You can have an orgasm and not be wet enough. You can be super horny and not get wet at all. It plays the biggest of big roles in quickies. Sometimes you're just like, "I need something in this vag, and I need it now." Lube is everything, and it helps bridge the barrier of different bodies and how they work. Every single body is different and reacts to stimuli differently. Lube, however, is always wet. Lube always lubricates.

Without lube, sex can get messy and not in a fun, sexy way . . . more like a bloody way. Skipping lube can cause vaginal tearing, and in case you were wondering, it's not fun. I was walking with a limp for a solid two days after the Halloween Weekend Dry Vagina Fiasco (trademark pending).

The last thing you want after a romp in the hay is the dire need to grab an ice pack for your coochie.

When it comes to all things sexual, from foreplay to fooling around to intercourse, the more drenched you can get your pussy, the better off your vagina (and clitoris and vulva) will be. It acts as a barrier to avoid unpleasant friction against the tender skin of the vagina and vulva. Your vulva is a special, magical place, and it needs to be treated with care. You wouldn't straighten your hair without using heat-protection spray, so why would you fuck without using some friction-protection lubricant? You wouldn't play field hockey without a guard to protect your teeth, so why would you have sex without something to protect your puss?

You know I was going to get to the butt stuff. You knew it was coming. If you want to do anything anal, you *need* lube. The asshole is a lovely, beautiful place full of many sexual possibilities, but it is as dry as a peach husk left out in the sun. Your butthole does not lubricate the same way a vagina does. It needs that good-ol' lube, kiddo. You need to make your dry asshole as slick as a waterslide.

Lube up your butt toys, lube up your fingers, lube up your penises, lube up your dildos. Lube, lube, and more lube.

A SLIPPERY BREAKDOWN: WHICH LUBE IS RIGHT FOR YOU?

Water-Based

Water-based lubes are my favorite. Go with 100 percent pure and organic lubes. Read the label. Be sure it doesn't contain glycerin, parabens, or petrochemicals. Studies have shown that shitty commercial brands like KY are full of chemicals that can throw off your vagina's pH, and glycerin can cause yeast infections. Try companies like Good Clean Love, Sustain Natural, and Babeland.

Silicone-Based

Silicone lube is the bomb because it stays on and never lets go. You don't have to reapply as much as a water-based. Be wary of use with condoms. Most silicone lubes are fine, but some have high oil contents and can damage the integrity of latex, causing breakage. Always Google the brand of lube and make sure it is latex-safe before using with condoms. Babeland, along with a few other companies, makes a hybrid silicone/water-based lube that won't damage condoms and stays put.

Silicone lube is especially useful during the butt brigade. When you're doing butt stuff, you need something that stays on since the anus is a supertight space with zero natural lubrication. Just be wary of the brand when using condoms (which should be always).

Silicone lube stains sheets and linens, so be careful. I am a lazy piece of shit, so in lieu of dealing with stains, I bought bright purple sheets so I wouldn't have to be bothered. On that note, don't come to my house with a black light, for the love of God.

Oil-Based Lube

Oil-based lubes are a decent choice if you and your partner are STI-free (again, problematic with the whole HPV thing). Oil-based lube cannot ever be used with condoms. Literally never. No. It damages latex and polyurethane, and your condoms will break.

The appeal? It stays on really well. Oil doesn't absorb into the skin the same way other lubes do, which means you're pretty slick for the whole ride. The thing that sucks most? Some kinds can throw off the pH of the vagina, causing infections or bacterial vaginosis (BV) in some women. Coconut oil, for example, is an antibacterial, which can kill good bacteria inside the vagina, making way for the overgrowth of bad bacteria.

Flavored Lubes

Speaking of bacterial vaginosis and yeast infections, do not put flavored lube in a vagina or on a vulva during oral or you will get BV or a yeast infection. They should go nowhere near your downstairs bits, Mama. Flavored lubes are sweet, which means they likely contain glycerin. Glycerin is a component found in sugar and will feed the natural yeast inside your vagina. Too much yeast leads to a yeast infection. Vaginas are interesting and weird. These lubes are full of artificial flavors. They are not a healthy option.

That being said, flavored lube makes blow jobs a lot more fun and appealing, and while they aren't good for your honeypot, they are safe for your mouth. Nothing makes you want to put a dick or dildo in your mouth like the promise of mint or strawberry.

Obviously, some flavored lubes are disgusting, but there are a few brands that make delicious options. Good Head is a solid choice. Just remember to wash off the lube completely before putting the penis/dildo/vibrator inside your vagina.

Warming Lubes

Be very careful with these kinds of lubes. You'll see labels that say, "Her pleasure," or "Clit-buzzing," or "Natural vibrating lube." Be wary.

Warming lubes were clearly created by someone without a vulva who thought they knew what women wanted. They can burn your clit/vagina off (not literally). If you have a sensitive vulva/vagina, these are not a good idea. I would recommend skipping them altogether if you're unsure about the product you're using. I'm a fan of Doc Johnson's clit-buzzing lube. This is the only one I have found that doesn't make my vulva feel like I doused it in cheap gin and lit a match. If we're being real, though, just don't use them on your vulva at all. There are other options. You don't need it.

All-Natural Lubes

Coconut Oil

Coconut oil is my personal favorite, but like I said, reports have shown the antibacterial properties can cause yeast infections for some women. If you're prone to the bread-baking life, skip this option. It's better to stick to a water-based organic lube if you've experienced BV or yeast infections in the past. Don't put weird shit in your cunt, because that never ends well.

Aloe Vera

And not that bullshit Banana Boat stuff. It needs to be 100 percent pure aloe vera. You can find it in Whole Foods or other natural grocery stores. I'm not sure if Wegman's, Jewel, or Costco has all-natural aloe. Ask a sales person. It's not like their mind would immediately go to: "This is FOR SURE being used for lube."

Almond Oil

Almond oil is legendary feminist queen and *Sex for One* author Betty Dodson's favorite lube. She swears by it, so I believe her. Almond oil doesn't have the same antibacterial properties of coconut oil, so you skip the risk of throwing off your pH. Make sure the almond oil you buy is 100 percent pure and doesn't contain any chemicals or outside ingredients.

HOW TO GET LUBED UP

There is nowhere you cannot apply lube. It can be applied liberally all over your and your partner's genitals.

Apply lube to your labia, clitoris, and sex toys before starting any sexual play. If your partner has a penis, apply lube generously to his (assuming he is male-identified) dick. Don't forget his balls, too!

Not everyone wants to have their balls played with, so make sure you know ahead of time if he enjoys having them played with before you go full monty.

You may not want to apply lube to your clitoris or labia before receiving oral sex. Some people don't enjoy the taste of lube. If you're using organic, natural options, you're probably fine (who doesn't love the taste of coconut?), but be sure to ask your partner before you go for it. All sexual pleasure is derived from asking for what you want and communicating effectively with your partner.

When it comes to good sex, don't skimp out on the stuff that makes it safer and better. You are a nasty woman who is in control of her sex life. Take precautions to make those experiences more fulfilling. You have the confidence and power to take control of your sexual excursions.

Don't put your safety or pleasure in the hands of another person. You know what feels good for your body, and you care about your body. Ask for what you want, and don't be afraid of getting shut down. Don't let anyone tell you that your personal agency isn't fucking beautiful and amazing. You are sexually empowered, and a sexually empowered woman doesn't have sex that doesn't feel good. That just isn't even worth it.

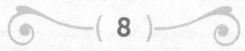

8

Gear Every Sexually Empowered Woman Needs to Have

When I was about eleven, well on my way into an early puberty, I discovered something very interesting—very interesting indeed. I spent a lot of time alone in my room giving myself hand jobs. As we already know, my longtime boyfriend (a.k.a. a bedpost) had shown me the glories of my nether regions. So at this point, I had been flicking my bean for a few years.

But I hadn't quite figured out yet that what I was doing was masturbation. I knew it felt good, so I kept on doing it. No self-control. It was a great secret to have. I didn't tell anyone about it. I didn't know it had anything to do with sex. I remember knowing that I had found out something very special about myself and figured no one else had this ability. I kind of felt like a secret agent because I had uncovered this miraculous thing that might be bad, but I figured if I didn't tell, no one would know. I had discovered all sorts of interesting ways to attain that feeling down below, the one that felt like sparks in my belly and crotchal region. Any chance I could get, I would do anything I could think of to make my clit buzz—hump the couch, hump my pillow, finger myself, grind against the zipper on my jeans—really anything.

Then everything changed. I found the all-powerful electric toothbrush in my bathroom. I don't know how I got the idea to use an electric toothbrush as a vibrator, but it turned out to be the first bootleg sex toy I ever owned—a starter vibe, if you will. I don't think it occurred to me that I had MacGyvered my own sex toy. I just thought I'd found a much easier solution to the carpal tunnel and wrinkly fingers I was experiencing from constantly smashing my clitoris. I was an engineer of sorts, a sexual pioneer attempting to maneuver my own body and growing horniness. I would take the head off the toothbrush and use the metal wand underneath to masturbate. I wrapped it in a shirt, because the metal rod was too strong to put directly on my clitoris. I would then rinse it and put the head back on. To be honest, I'm not 100 percent sure it was my toothbrush. If I had to guess, I would say it was one of my brothers'. This information makes me uncomfortable because it is gross. I also don't care because I am gross.

My second vibe, many years later, was a ginormous diva-white, incredibly phallic, rhinestone-encrusted knockoff Rabbit. I had seen the Rabbit in that famous episode of *Sex and the City* wherein Charlotte swears off men in favor of the guaranteed orgasm only her vibrator can provide. That Rabbit became the center of many an adolescent wish list. Mine was not the real Rabbit, though the genuine item is pretty aggressive, too. Mine was straight-up trash. It was '90s Britney Spears if Britney were a sex toy and somehow also made of rubber and/or jelly and/or nightmares. This vibrator was the scariest sex toy I had ever seen, but somehow very liberating. It made me feel very adult. At twenty-one, I would use it in my lofted bed in the three-bedroom apartment I shared with two gay men and a straight guy, clown car-style, on the Upper West Side.

It was a symbol of my maturation—the first adult toy I owned as an almost-adult. I held on to that piece of shit until I moved into an apartment in the East Village with my (now ex) long-term boyfriend at twenty-five.* Like an old friend, it came along with me, long after it had retired, from apartment to apartment for four whole years. We had good times, that piece-of-shit Rabbit and me.

Think about your first sex toy (assuming you've had one—because as we know, nearly half of women have never had one). What are your feelings about that toy? What was your experience buying it? If you've never had a vibrator, that's fine, too. If you finish reading this book and don't go buy some sex toys, I'm going to be mad at you, though. I'm petty like that, as we've established. All those memes about being "petty AF"—those are about me. Don't fuck with me. Go buy yourself some sex toys, you sexy bitch.

There are certain things every single sexually empowered woman needs to have to learn about her body and find out what she likes. If you're a sex-positive female, you need to take your pleasure into your own hands by buying the right stuff for *you*. If, like, you want to buy cock rings or whatever for your partner, that's cool, but start with the self-centered shit first. What stuff do you need, you ask? Right this way.

WHY SEX TOYS ARE IMPORTANT FOR WOMEN EVERYWHERE

Let me just say, hail to the finger. Your fingers are dope. You can do a lot with those dexterous phalanges. They are your first built-

---

* At twenty-five, three years feels very, very long-term.

in sex toy. Between your fingers and the bathtub faucet (don't even play, you know what I'm talking about), discovering your body is exciting and weird. Exploring your body helps you learn what you like and how you want to be touched by a partner(s). If you know how you like your clit touched, you will know how to tell a partner to touch you.

Exploring first with your fingers is a great way to go, but it can get exhausting to rub your clit. It becomes tedious and a little boring. I have a weak right wrist. Like, problems-doing-cartwheels-and-planks-level weak. I'm convinced that shit is from the right-handed hand jobs that colored my youth. Carpal tunnel, man. The struggle is real. I mean, tired hands and wrists were the reason men invented vibrators in the first place.

Strap on your seat belts, because here is a brief history lesson. You're welcome. Don't act like you don't want to know how the Magic Wand became a thing. Spoiler: It wasn't because people wanted women to have orgasms and control over their sexual well-being. It was because women were interested in sexual pleasure, and this was something men couldn't control. You can trust me on this because a) I'm amazing and b) I thoroughly researched this shit for *Elle* one time.

The vibrator was developed in 1869 (the immature hilarity of the 69 is not lost on me) by the physician George Taylor. Doctors in the Victorian era were basically jacking women off to cure "hysteria." They thought that women were high-strung and mentally ill, just because we had feelings about shit. It is an entirely made-up illness. Straight-up bullshit. It does not exist.

You might be wondering, *What the hell do you mean there was a made-up illness created by confused and idiotic doctors who then chose to rub one out for women everywhere?* When men can't figure something out or experience it for themselves, they slap a tag on it and wash their hands (pun intended) of the whole thing. It's a lot like postpartum depression, or menopause, or being an intellectual, complex thinker about things other than baked goods: Men don't experience these things, so they make up reasons for why it's happening. And—big shocker—they are fucking wrong a lot. Hysteria turned out to just be sexual frustration and a general capacity for emotions. Not having orgasms will literally drive you bonkers.

It was widely believed in the western Victorian world that women didn't experience sexual pleasure at all. The female orgasm was not something that was looked into. People were like, "Sex is for making babies, and men are the only ones who like it," and women were over here like, "Um. Hello? Actually, never mind— we're busy trying not to be thrown in a mental institution for having an original thought." Not fucking around. This happened a lot. Some women loved having orgasms so much that they kept making appointments and would come in regularly for their "treatments." Hi? Hello? Women love coming.

Let's be clear here—someone rubbing your clitoris to make you orgasm without consent is sexual assault—even in a clinical setting. It doesn't matter if a doctor thinks making you come your face off is a "cure." No one can touch you without your a) being aware of what the actual hell is happening, as women of the time didn't, and b) without your desire to be touched in this way, for sexual reasons.

You know what was actually happening? People didn't know a clitoris was for pleasure. Women weren't getting clitoral stimulation during sex (remember how the full structure of the clitoris was discovered in the 1990s? Good times) and therefore weren't orgasming. Meanwhile, all these dudes were like, "This is hard! My hands are tired from rubbing so many clitorises!!!" Lo and behold, the birth of the vibe. The crackhead men of medicine invented vibrators so they could calm hysteria without getting carpal tunnel. Clearly, the 1800s had no chill.

WHY ALL FEMINISTS SHOULD INVEST IN SEX TOYS

Over time, sex toys went from being purely medical devices, to being disguised as personal massagers, to actually being called what they were: fucking sex toys. Thank for the vibes, Doc. I got this now. Bye. I am the queen of my clit, bye-bye. *Bye.*

Despite its roots, the vibrator is now the sword we wield in our act of resistance. We don't need another person to make us feel good, and that is liberating AF.

Now, before you go screaming, *"Misandrist!"* at me (trust me, the Twitter trolls have beaten you to it), it's not to say that you don't want a partner (male or female or nonbinary or genderqueer, etc., etc.). Falling in love is awesome, and if you want to be with someone, that's incredible and I am so happy for you. But knowing you don't need another person to make yourself come is important and crucial to your confidence and self-worth. As a sex-positive, feminist, badass bitch, you need to take your pleasure into your own hands. You need to know what you like, how to get it, and how to ask for it. Only then will you be on your way to demanding a life and relationship that is worthy of you. You can want a partner, but you don't need one. You are complete and perfect on your own.

Sex toys are tools to explore your body and learn what it likes. It is a feminist proclamation of self to have a great sex toy collection. It says, "I don't care what you think of me or my sexuality because I am in control and do with it as I please." Fuck the haters. Your sex toy collection is an empowering symbol of your freedom and choice. Own it. Live it.

A vibrator is something every single woman should have. If it were up to me (Gigi for president 2020??), girls would be given vibrators by their moms. Yeah, a vibrator in the hands of every female. That's the America I want to see. There is nothing wrong with masturbating, and we should be encouraging girls to do it. We should look at both young women (and young men) and be able to recognize and celebrate that this child is a sexual being.

If you know how to get off, you're way less likely to go poking around the schoolyard for a boy or girl to do it for you. This is one of the many, many reasons why so many girls have sex before they're ready; they think it's going to be the answer to their horniness. It isn't. Give a girl a sex toy and she can rule the world. Shaming your kid into thinking her body is nasty and gross does not foster a strong, self-sufficient adult. If you start a girl off thinking her body is a beautiful, magical beacon of wonder and she should know all about it, how it works, and what makes it feel good—you can bet your ass she's much less likely to let some idiot fuck with her life. All this from a vibrator. The Excalibur of pussy whispering. God bless America. Amen.

Fine, y'all. I'm finished with the tirade. Let's get back to shit you need to invest in. Treat your pussy/body like a 14-karat gold, ruby-encrusted, Hope Diamond–ass-level prize.

SEX TOYS GO BEYOND VIBRATORS

Word up. There is no limit to the gear you can buy. After that masturbation, clitastic chapter you read before this, you know that self-
exploration is the stuff of life, and you should venture wherever
your ~~heart~~ clit desires. If you're just starting your sex toy collection,
there are a few key things every sex-positive woman should keep in
her boudoir (or wherever you're fucking or masturbating because
you get to choose, Mama).

Clit toys: If you're buying your first sex toy and don't know where
to begin, get a clit vibe. Sex toy websites have sections designated
for your clitoris.

These are small, often adorable vibrators and are not at all scary.
Some toys even look like lipsticks or the eggplant emoji—no joke,
I used it, and it's pretty rad. They can either be battery operated or
recharged via USB, depending on the one you choose. These are
your basic starter vibes, but they can also be used during sex for
clit stimulation. You can take them with you anywhere because
they are easily stored in a purse or backpack. Next time you have a
Tinder fuck, you've got a friend to come along with you.

Butt toys: Anal play is amazing, and you do not need a prostate to
enjoy it. Most of the nerves in the entire ass are clustered in the
opening of the anus—meaning most of the feeling and pleasure
will be felt right there in the first couple of inches. Butt plugs are
exactly what they sound like—a plug for the butthole. They come
with either a flared base or a ring on the end. You don't want to put
anything up your ass without a flared base. A common miscon-

ception: *Oh, I'll just poop it out if it gets lost.* Nope. Not a thing. You could wind up with an obstructed bowel if you shove something not made for an ass up your ass. Be careful and always follow the directions. Oh, and lube. Lots of lube.

I. Butt plugs:

Start small. I mean, really small. Like, the smallest one you can find. I once got a medium-size butt plug thinking that I wore medium-size shirts so I was a medium in everything. Same thing, right? Not the same thing. You need to work up to bigger toys. Your butthole is a muscle, and its natural inclination is to push out. Lube the butt plug up with an all-natural organic lubricant (jump to chapter 7 really quickly if you're curious about lube). Massage the butt and relax before insertion.

II. Vibrators for the butt:

Yes, these exist and are wonderful. There are quite a few companies that make a lot of awesome vibrators for your derrière. The nerve-rich opening of the anus really benefits from vibration.

G-spot toys: Your G-spot, as we've previously discussed, is located inside the vagina. It is still a part of the clitoris: the internal portion. It's more of an area than actual spot. It surrounds the urethral sponge and varies in size. The G-spot is the root of the clitoris, and you're accessing it from inside. To find it, insert two fingers into the vagina and make a hook, or a "come hither" motion. Behind the pubic bone, you'll feel a walnut-textured patch. It may also extend beyond this. This is the G-spot. It's different for everyone, but when stimulated, it feels like warm water washing over my whole vulva. It's like my pussy is singing that one song by Dave Matthews Band if Dave Matthews Band weren't shitty.

G-spot wands are sometimes curved, sometimes straight toys designed to reach this area of the internal clit. When you think of a wand, you may first imagine one of the dildo-type vibes that look like dicks (much like my trash-Rabbit. RIP). While these exist and are easy to find, they do not make up the whole or even the majority of G-spot wands available to you, my little magical unicorn baby.

For many a vulva owner, a dick-like G-spot wand is *not* attractive. This may apply especially to a vulva owner who prefers sex with other vulva owners, but it's definitely not an exclusively queer phenomenon. Even the dick-loving among us might be anti-dick when it comes to the wand.

My favorite wands are curved like a bow for easy access to the area behind the pubic bone. I'm not trying to fuck around when it comes to getting at my hot spots. Wands come in all shapes and sizes, but you don't need to buy something the size of a tree trunk. These toys are diverse. You can use them for solo-clit action, G-spot stimulation, or with a partner for clit stimulation. Because they are generally pretty sizable, and some come with a handle, they are choice for reaching the clitoris in more dexterous sexual positions like doggy-style or spooning.

Couple's vibe: Fewer than 30 percent of women can orgasm through intercourse alone, so what the actual fuck are we doing having sex without toys? Now, you can use your fingers if you want to do that. It's chill. Obviously, you can do whatever the fuck you want, but a sex toy is the helping hand we all need. If the Hamburger Helper Hand were actually legit, he'd vibrate. (Is that joke too old for you?)

These small, inconspicuous sex toys are fabulous additions to your sex life. Trying to explain how this shit works to my mother was frustrating.

> Mom: *You wear it* during *sex? But how? How does that work if the penis goes into you??*
> Me: *You hook it to either inside the labia, or one end goes into the vagina and the other over the clitoris.*
> Mom:
> Me:
> Mom: *What?*
> Me: *Read the directions. There are pictures.*
> Mom: *???*

Toys like Eva (and Eva II) from Dame and the We-Vibe Sync can be worn during sex to offer clitoral stimulation during intercourse. It takes the pressure off your partner to make you come from penetration and allows you to get off without a shitload of extra work. It's a win-win for everyone.

It doesn't matter if you're single, dating someone, fucking everyone, or married; you should have a couple's vibe in your collection. You should feel empowered to bring it out on a one-night stand and get off. Why the hell would you not? You signed up for an orgasm, and if you need a toy to get off, you should be entitled to use one. If a person isn't comfortable with that, do you really want to have sex with them?

If a guy or girl you're with says you can't use sex toys but isn't willing to get his or her fingers/mouth up in there to do what it takes to ensure that you have a satisfying sexual experience, that isn't someone you should be fucking.

Life is too short for bad sex and bullshit people. Everyone not only deserves to have an orgasm during sex, it's a goddamn right.

No, but like, Gigi, what do I buy? The options are overwhelming me.

Honey, you never looked better.

DON'T BUY GROSS SHIT: KNOWING YOUR MATERIALS

Seriously, do not buy gross shit. Some sex toys are made from low-grade, piece-of-shit materials, and you really don't need that in your life or anywhere near your cunt. If I had known how disgusting that white Rabbit actually was, I would have thrown up on myself. It was partially made of jelly, a porous material that holds bacteria and can never be properly cleaned. It can never be disinfected. If you use a badly made toy, there will always be germies hiding in the crevices of your toy. There will be crusted pussy juices you can never liberate. That's nasty as fuck and not in a good way. In the literal definition way.

A problem worth noting, sex toys and adult pleasure products aren't subjected to much (if any) scrutiny by the FDA. There is, like, no regulation. This is pretty fucked up. Like, imagine if your beef wasn't regulated by the FDA and farmers could just give you whatever meat they wanted without worrying about getting in trouble. Adult pleasure companies are not forced to adhere to any rules when it comes to making toys safe for the body and not out of materials that are shitty. This is, in a word, fucked. We put a lot of sex toys inside of and outside of our bodies and don't know if they're safe. So, to do due diligence, you need to be careful about what you buy. I know it feels like a scam, and that's because it is a scam. We should have standards for this shit, but adult toys are so highly stigmatized in this culture that we can't even get the FDA to give a fuck. Meanwhile, everyone is buying and using sex toys—even the people in the FDA, probably.

Reading the Directions

Always read the fucking directions. I know it's tedious and boring. Listen, I get it. You don't want to pull out that tiny stupid manual (ew, is this Calibri font?) when you just got a new orgasm-giving toy. Buying a new sex toy is really exciting, and I'm so happy for you. It's a beautiful moment in time, and bountiful orgasms await you. This doesn't mean you should just go forth without knowing what the fuck you're doing. It's not like you had a class on how to use adult products in school. You have to self-educate. Sex toys come in all shapes, sizes, and functionalities. Does your toy have a motor? Is it made of porous material? All of these details are going to dictate how you clean and maintain your sex toys. Like, sex toys are expensive, so you need to know how to take care of them.

Knowing Your Materials

1. **JELLY:** This is an absolute no-no. It's a porous material and holds bacteria. Some really shitty sex toy shops will have cock rings, masturbation sleeves, and vile vibrators made from horrifying, cheap materials. Jelly is the stuff of nightmares.
   How to clean it: Throw it in the fucking garbage. Light it on fire if you want, but actually don't because fumes.

2. **ELASTOMER AND CYBERSKIN:** A cousin of jelly, these are better but imperfect choices. Both are still slightly porous, so

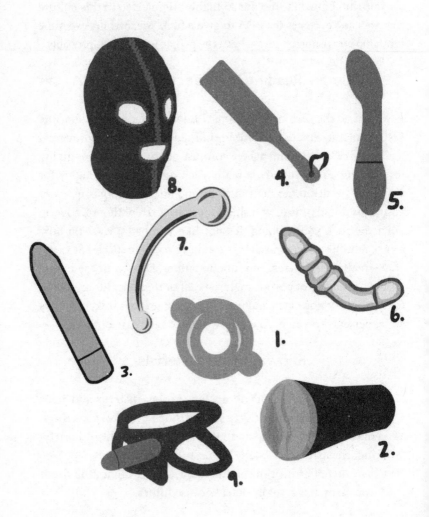

disinfecting is more difficult than harder materials. There is an appeal of elastomer for toys like Fleshlights and masturbation sleeves (for people with penises), because it has a soft, pleasant texture. It feels a lot like a real vagina or anus.

Elastomer is sometimes used with certain vibrators and can deliver those vibrations in a lovely way, especially for those who have sensitive clitorises. It acts like a barrier in the way my T-shirt used to when I jacked myself off with a toothbrush.

How to clean it: You can use a gentle soap and water to wash it. Then leave it on a clean towel to fully dry. Keep in mind that it won't be completely disinfected because it technically can never be fully cleaned. A great option: Get a UV sex toy cleaning box. These are boxes full of UV lights that kill bacteria on your sex toys. It's like a tanning bed, only not horrible for you. They won't remove all the bacteria, but they'll help. For toys made of these materials, don't use them with multiple partners, as you can't fully clean them and could spread infections.

3. **HARD PLASTIC:** Hard plastic is a great choice. Make sure it is ABA designated. This is how you know for sure that it's nonporous. It can be 100 percent disinfected. It has a sleek, hard texture so it can really get in the butthole and reach the G-spot. Materials like hard plastic: ceramic and Lucite.

How to clean it: A mild soap and water will do the trick. Always use something unscented, as the chemicals in scented soaps can irritate vulva skin. You can also get a disinfecting sex toy spray for easy and quick cleanups. Just be sure it's a spray that doesn't use a lot of harsh chemicals. Buy one from your local sex toy boutique and check the ingredients. Stay away from store-brand shit like Windex. Despite what you heard in *My Big Fat Greek Wedding,* it really is not a cure-all for everything.

4. **WOOD:** Most wooden sex toys (paddles, G-spot wands, canes, etc.) are coated in a layer of polyurethane or a lacquer that is body-safe. This makes it waterproof. Sometimes, these coats can wear down over time, which means your toy can become porous. Be sure to keep a close eye on the directions and ask a sex toy salesperson what the wood is coated in.

How to clean it: Soap and water will do just fine. Set it out on a dry, clean towel, and let it thoroughly dry out before using again. You can also use alcohol or diluted bleach (follow the directions for diluting bleach on the back of the bottle). Rinse thoroughly with water to avoid harsh chemicals making contact with your vulva.

5. **SILICONE:** If you can stick with a toy that is 100 percent silicone, go for it. Silicone toys are my absolute favorite. You know what you're getting and don't have to freak out about germs and bacteria.

Many companies will say their silicone is "body-safe," but this is misleading. The only body-safe silicone is medical-grade silicone. If it says *medical grade,* you are in the clear. This is totally an advertising plug, so if a company uses medical-grade silicone, they will want you to know. There are companies that are all about your safety (ahem, companies founded and run by women who actually know what it takes to have a healthy vag).

How to clean: Soap and water, baby. If the toy doesn't have a motor, you can put it in the dishwasher or pop it in a pot of boiling water to disinfect.

6. **GLASS:** LOL, did you just say *glass?* Yeah, boo, there are toys made of glass. You do have to be gentle with them. Don't use them if they're chipped. Don't use it if you dropped it and think it *might* be chipped. Glass toys, like Babeland's G-Spot wands, are fucking works of art. You've seen those dudes on Venice Beach who blow their own glass pipes with designs and colors galore? These wands are just like that. They are magical. Fuck collecting art. You should collect glass dildos. Dildos are as beautiful as sexual empowerment itself, I'm telling you. You might be thinking, *Why the actual fuck would I put a glass dildo in my pussy?* The answer is: The weight feels amazing on your G-spot and/or clitoris.

How to clean: Most glass toys are top-rack dishwasher safe, but I'd suggest boiling them. If they have a fancy design, the dishwasher could potentially screw them up. I might be paranoid about this one, but better safe than sorry. They are so pretty, you don't want to fuck them up.

7. **STAINLESS STEEL:** Stainless steel toys are heavy and wonderful for G-spot and anal stimulation. They're kind of kinky, which is pretty sexy. They are metal, and metal is kind of dangerous and, um, metal. Nothing says you're in control and love to get down like a curved, steel, rigged G-spot wand. Excuse me, I need a napkin to wipe my seat up.

How to clean: I love a good stainless steel sex toy because you can boil that shit in a pot or pop it in the dishwasher and you are good to go.

8. **LEATHER:** Leather is primarily used for harnesses (for strap-ons, swings, etc.), crops, masks, and so on. A regular vibrator

or sex toy probably won't be made of leather. It's a kinky material and is super fierce. I recommend everyone have at least a riding crop in her possession, if only to know it is there.

How to clean: Leather is porous and can't be fully disinfected. Your UV light box can help, but it won't fully do the job. You can use leather cleaner to shine and wipe it down. If you're using leather equipment, it's better to use different stuff for each partner. I know it's expensive, but leather is an investment.

9. NYLON AND SPANDEX: Nylon and spandex are used primarily for harnesses and other wearable gear like costumes (cotton is also a material used in role play). It's something to be aware of since you may very well get them covered in bodily excretions and lube.

How to clean: Pop them in the washing machine with your towels. Let both materials air-dry. You don't want to wind up with a naughty nurse costume two sizes too small after a run in the drier. Not sexy.

BASIC MAINTENANCE 101

The Hot-Pink Rule: Do Not Cross-Pollinate Your Sex Toys

Keep your butt toys and your vag toys separate. Silicone and stainless steel can be the exception, provided they are boiled and washed beforehand. The last thing you need is fecal matter getting anywhere near your vulva or vagina. That is a yeast infection / bacterial vaginosis / toxic shock waiting to happen.

Listen, a lot of peeps will tell you it's okay to put a silicone toy up your cunt, post–butt stuff, if you've washed it thoroughly, but that is not a risk I'm willing to take. A sex toy collection should have plenty of stuff and lots of variety. You can get things for your butt and things for your vagina/clit and call it a day. Follow the hot-pink rule so that you don't run into any unwanted, super-awkward trips to the ob-gyn/ER. Personally, I don't want to explain to a broad-shouldered nurse named Cassandra that I may have accidentally put poop up my vagina. Call me crazy.

True story, though, speaking of poop up vaginas. I had this terrible, abusive, psycho ex-boyfriend when I was in my very early twenties. He was in his late thirties, which only makes what I'm about to tell you even more unacceptable and obvious that we need better, more comprehensive sex ed in schools.

I had just finished my period the day before, and we were getting it on. We were in doggy-style when suddenly he pulled out and said, "There is fecal matter all over my cock." Now, that is probably the stupidest way to say *I have poop on my dick* that I have ever heard (*Fecal matter?* Seriously? Is it 1879?), but that's not really the point. He looked at me with such disgust. I, being a twenty-year-old with limited self-confidence and understanding of my own body, became flustered and embarrassed. I got dressed and left his apartment immediately. He made no attempt to stop me.

Once I got down on the street and had a moment to process what had happened, it all made sense. I didn't have shit up my vagina. You can't just get poop up your vagina. I would probably have been in the hospital if by some strange fluke in anatomy I was able to stick shit up my cunt.

It was oxidized blood. I had just finished up my menses. Blood turns brown when it is exposed to oxygen. It was just some leftover fucking period blood. A thirty-seven-year-old man thought he had shit dick and had apparently never seen a period. I can't. I texted him. He didn't respond. We never spoke of it again because that's what mature adults do, duh.*

CLEAN YOUR TOYS EVERY SINGLE TIME YOU USE THEM

Do not just let the crust sit and fester. You have to clean your toys every single time you use them, thoroughly. It is not up for negotiation. If you use unclean sex toys, you can wind up getting bacterial vaginosis or another vaginal infection. It's not a good idea, and it is unsanitary and gross.

You don't have to pop up after a hot love fest and be like, "BRB, boo! Gotta pop this dildo in a boiling pot!" Just put them aside, in a place where you can get to them later. Get a designated tray or bin for dirty sex toys, one where you can throw your used toys to clean later.

DON'T SUBMERGE TOYS WITH MOTORS IN WATER

If your toy has a motor or motors, you cannot boil it or submerge it in water. Use mild antibacterial soap and water to clean the toy. You can get it wet, but do not drop it in a pot or filled sink.

---

* Didn't break up with him, though. He was rich, and I was way too poor to give that shit up. Normal!

How do you know if it has a motor? Does it move, vibrate, jiggle, and so on? If yes, it has a motor. Read the directions that come with the toy and be sure you know how to clean it before you go fucking around with it.

Some toys, even ones without motors, aren't suitable for soaking (like some wooden toys, as it may damage them). Always follow the directions.

STORE YOUR SEX TOYS IN A CLEAN, DRY PLACE

Last but not least, store your sex toys in a clean, dry spot where they won't collect bacteria or dust. Make sure they are completely dry before storing. Don't throw sex toys in the bottom of a plastic bin under the bed and leave them there to rot. A panty drawer or night table is fine. You can also invest in a storage box.

A local sex toy boutique will have all kinds of options for sex toy storage. You can hit up your local Bed Bath & Beyond if you want something that thoroughly blends in with your décor.*

Whatever you choose to buy, make sure it's stuff that suits your own sexual curiosities. You don't have to buy everything I've listed; these are just suggestions to help you get started. Sex toys are a rad way to figure out what you want to try and explore. Enjoy yourself. They aren't called *toys* for nothing.

---

* You know what they say—if your sex toy storage is luxe, you are wife material. It's a real saying. It is.

WHERE TO SHOP: THE GLORIES OF FEMINIST SEX TOY STORES

Now, I'm sure you're like, *OMG, yas! I want all of these toys. I want five of each. Where do I buy them? Because I'm not trying to go into some creepy fucking store where a chubby dude with plumber's crack gives me side-eye in a hella creepy but somehow also super-judgmental way.*

Oh, girl. I know. When it comes down to shopping for a dildo, a vibrator, or whatever it is you're looking for, the shopping experience is one of the biggest hurdles.

I remember my first year in New York when I found my way into a sex shop in the West Village on Christopher Street. There were half-naked mannequins in the window and rows and rows of adult DVDs. A lighted sign flashed on and off reading, "Peep Shows!" I was with a few of my friends. We wandered around like your typical nineteen-year-old asshats, giggling over purple dildos and cheap polyester strap-ons.

Sex shops didn't really get much better the older I got. Years later, I found myself buying a jelly (jelly, so gross) cock ring with my then partner in what I imagine was the seediest shop in Ithaca, New York. The cock ring (*fucking jelly*) wound up covered in lint and was way stickier than it should have been. It was fun for, like, a weekend. It turned my ex boyfriend's wang into a vibrator, and I was about it, but we threw that fucker right in the garbage before trekking back to the city in our rental car.

Sometimes you want a quick cock ring disco stick ride and need to buy a piece of shit jelly toy from the Dollar Store Dildo Super Emporium. It happens to the best of us. YOLO. Regardless of life's hiccups, don't make these trash piles the places you regularly go.

You get to avoid all those horrible, germ-filled, crappily made toys if you shop in the right places. The right places do, indeed, exist. You don't even have to go a brick-and-mortar-style shop, my friend. All of the best shops have online stores. You can shop for G-spot wands and clit vibes in the comfort of your bathrobe.

FEMINIST SEX TOY STORES ARE EVERYWHERE

There are many more, but some of my favorite places to shop are: Babeland, Please, Good Vibrations, SheBop, SheVibe, Come as You Are, the Pleasure Chest, and Early to Bed.

These stores are the best because they are designed to make shopping for sex toys a happy, pleasant, shame-free experience. They are stores founded by women for women. The aesthetics are super pleasing—like, everything is pink and silky and fabulous—but not in an over-the-top pseudo "girly" way. It's warm, inviting, and super sex-positive. Sex shouldn't be this shameful thing, and exploring your body should be encouraged. These stores help you feel good about your decision to have a fun and fulfilled sex life. It's kind of like being in one of those Japanese Hello Kitty cafés mixed with a high-end shoe store.

The staff is trained to answer every single question you might have. Nothing you ask is stupid. Nothing you want to know is off limits. These are people who want to help you. They are happy and overjoyed that you are here to explore your sexual pleasure. They will make you feel like a goddamn clit queen. Everyone is so nice, so knowledgeable, and so friendly. They will make sure you find toys as unique as you are. I'm not even joking.

When people with vaginas make toys for people with vaginas, you get shit that is actually good and a shopping experience that makes you comfortable and at home rather than skeeved the fuck out.

I could write a million love notes to my collection of sex toys, the beautiful woman-friendly boutiques where I've shopped, and the wonderful people who helped me find my soul mate dildos. There are no words that can properly thank them for all the joy they have brought to my life. The Patriarchy would like to think that what we ladies value most are shoes and clothes. Now, shoes and clothes are amazing, don't get me wrong, but for a sexually empowered woman, shoes ain't got nothin' on sex toys.

Have a conversation with the person (or people) you are sleeping with about sex toys. Don't be afraid to talk about what you like and what you need in bed. You want this person to know where you're coming from and to understand your sexual proclivities. Listen to what they have to say as well. Be open to hearing them out. Sex is only truly amazing when both people are getting what they want out of the experience.

If you find people in your life who aren't down with your love of orgasms and dildos du jour, don't hang out with those people anymore. If you took the time to have an adult conversation and they're still being a douchelord about it, get the hell out of there.

The older you get, the more you realize that people are by and large the worst. Stick with your sex-positive, supportive tribe and suit up against the world. This is just a friendly reminder that you do not have to keep people in your life who make you feel badly about yourself, your desires, or your body. You are not obligated to stay friends with assholes.

Oh, one last thing—a tip I wish I had had so many times I could scream. Most toys with motors come with chargers. All the chargers somehow look the same and always get lost. Get a bucket so you can keep all your sex toy chargers in one place. Every toy has a different cord, and they will go missing. Trust me, I'm saving you a lot of time.*

Now, go forth and unsheathe your metaphorical sword and come your face off, queen. You've got the info you need to get the tools you want . . . and the sex you deserve.

---

* I had to ask Dame Products to send me a new charger one time. They did it, which was so chill.

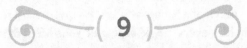

Can You Send a Text About Choking on a Cock and Still Be a Feminist?

To answer that question: Yes. You totally can want to choke on a cock, feel balls on your chin, be neck-deep in a pussy, suck a clit, get spanked, indulge in a consensual rape (*ravishment,* if you prefer) fantasy, and get fucked against a door and still be a feminist. So get the fucking dumb AF ideas out of your head that you can't love dick, puss, or both and still want gender equality.

And when it comes to texting about it, you should absolutely be able to get your freak on via text without feeling like a psycho / liar / bad feminist / whore. Let's stop being shitheads about this. A feminist can be (in real life and on a mobile phone, with or without emojis) a submissive, she can love pussy, she can love being slapped in the face with a dick, she can want a dick up her ass. *Want* is the key word here. If you're doing something you want to do and feel in control, you are doing something feminist. If you were being forced to do this or coerced, or were engaging in this behavior to please someone, that would be fucked up.

A nasty woman has a way with most words, but often sexting

and dirty talk can be intimidating. Performance anxiety is real, no matter how much of a badass you are. It's pretty hard to be a stone-cold bad bitch in every single aspect of your life. For many of us, sexting or dirty talk is a pain point.

Sexting is an art we all can master. It allows us to explore fantasy in a safe and secure way, giving us a chance to test the waters on something we may not be totally comfortable with yet—whether it be bondage, anal, or whatever. I'm going to hold your hand and help you figure out what kind of sexter you are, how to get started, the easiest way to transfer those writing skills into dirty talk, and, finally, a ton of exercises to hone your skills.

Listen, one of my favorite workshops I teach is a sexting 101 class. It's mostly bachelorette parties and middle-aged women who sign up, and I'm totally fine with that. It's also BYOB so, you know, shit gets weird.

I started teaching after doing a lot of learning myself. This is something I needed practice with. I went to a bunch of workshops about dirty talk and bedroom communication, something that I objectively sucked at doing for a long time.

I'd now classify myself as a porn star–level sexter.

When I was in my last relationship (like the one before I met my husband), I found that I was regularly running out of things to say in the sack. You can only tell your boyfriend how sexy and hard he is so many times before it becomes boring, you know? You can only tell your girlfriend how wet her pussy is for you before you're like, "KK. Dope. Now what?"

One night in November of 2016, with an open mind and reasonable level of anxiety, I made the journey uptown to Thirty-fourth Street in Manhattan for a dirty-talking class.

The class was held in a Midtown audition studio, the stomping ground for aspiring Broadway actors. The sound of a grand piano and off-key singing echoed throughout the space. Incidentally, I don't like theater people because they are all kinds of terrible (sorry if you're a theater person; I'm sure you're great).

Despite the high energy that comes with theater hopefuls, there was something oddly appropriate about the location. Talking dirty definitely requires some acting, exuberance, and a positive attitude. Most of us don't wander around using dirty talk in everyday conversation, so talking dirty without it seeming ridiculous requires checking your inhibitions and adopting a different persona. Luckily, our studio was tucked away in the back so as not to draw too much attention to the fact we were there learning how to describe our cunts with ferocious adjectives and adverbs.

My class, hosted by StripXpertease, consisted of four ladies seated around a big plastic table in a glorified ballet studio, ready to get nasty for fifty-two dollars a pop.

What I loved most was how kind and nonjudgmental everyone was. It felt good to be surrounded by supportive women. After completing and reading our workbook exercises aloud, we went around the room and read a porn scene together. I didn't laugh once. I didn't even feel (that) awkward. We all wanted to expand our dirty-talk vocabularies and upgrade our bedroom skills.

I learned a lot in my two-hour workshop that night, including new internal question marks around certain "sexy" terms, such as *meat curtains* and *sperminator*. Were these actual words people used? I shuddered, imagining a partner saying, "I'm going to pierce your meat curtains with my sperminator."

I walked out of class feeling strong and empowered. My partner at the time probably could have done without the amount of times I said *hard cock* and *pussy* on the F train that night, but he was happy to see me so full of life and excited about something. You see, sexting and dirty talk aren't something you just magically know how to do. So if you think you're somehow broken because you don't know how to accurately describe or feel comfortable with telling someone to come on your face, that's okay.

Sexting is a little like porn; it's a fantasy. I love texting my sex partners extremely graphic fantasies about how I want them to fill me up in every hole and come all over my body. Meanwhile, I mostly have fairly "regular" sex and only do butt stuff on occasion.

Technology has made all of this wonderment and fantasy possible. I mean, sexting is a relatively new thing. People have been sending dirty love letters since the invention of the written word, but sexting was born out of technology. Once we had instant messaging, we had sexting. Relatively speaking to, you know, the history of the world, it's brand spankin' new. Meaning, no one knows what the fuck they're doing.

Cell phones and IM-ing sent our sex lives into the ether, making it possible to drag out foreplay over an entire day at the office. At the same time, you don't want to freak anyone out over sext, you know? There is always worry over whether or not you've crossed a line. You know what I mean, girl. That eerily painful ". . ." response bubble could run you emotionally ragged.

Should I not have told her I wanted to suck her clit until she was begging for more? Should I have skipped the part where I suggested he toss my salad like a whirlwind?

More than that, it's confusing when the person you're texting sends you something fucking gnarly and you're not down. Which begs the question: If you're sexually empowered, shouldn't everything go? No. *Nope.* That's canceled.

We'll get to all of that because a smart, luscious woman like you should be able to get her sexting jollies without feeling weird about it.

Then, of course, comes the even harder part: transferring all of that nasty text into talk. Hence why I took a class on this. I've gotten better, by the way. I'll share some secrets my instructor definitely did not teach me but should have.

Spoken-word dirty talk can be intimidating and downright awkward AF. I remember one of my friends came to me after the first time hooking up with someone and told me he kept telling her to talk dirty to him. It made her so uncomfortable she not only said nothing but she made no noise whatsoever. She lay there like a paralyzed jellyfish for the rest of the sexual encounter.

SEXTING: THE BASICS

So, like, let's talk about the sexting basics because where the actual fuck do you even start? It's not like you're going to jump right into a flirtatious text exchange with the hot girl you met on Bumble only to say, "I want you to touch my butthole."

Butthole text not (necessarily) included, sexting should be fun. It's perfectly acceptable to laugh (the other person can't even see you). It's okay to feel nervous before you send something dirty. We need to acknowledge how awkward sexting is. Yes, it can be mad awkward. If we did more to accept the awkwardness and move into a frame of mind where people didn't feel like pervs for sexting, everyone would be doing more, healthy sexting. Obviously, this goes back to all the shame we have surrounding sex. No one knows how to talk about sex, so we all feel weird about sex in any and all forms.

Rule #1 of getting on with your bad self is: Don't take yourself so seriously. When you treat sexting like a senior thesis or a spinal tap, it stops being fun. If it's not fun, you are not going to enjoy doing it. Sexting is a good place to explore things outside of your box (or inside of your other box, if you know what I mean). If it makes you feel anxious or vile, think of it as a brain exercise. That's what always helps me. You're essentially challenging yourself to come up with creative ways to describe things and increase your language skills and aptitude for metaphor. Ideally, you can then shift your focus to how hot sexting can be at some point. Sexting takes practice. The more you do it, the less uncomfortable it gets—just like masturbating, blow jobs, sex, and everything else.

Sexting is boundaryless, which can be confusing. How do you know *when* to send the sext or when to not send the sext? Sexting plays best in a variety of different kinds of relationships from the very serious, to the Tinder or Bumble hookup. It fully depends on who you are and what you like doing. If you want to save sexting for your boyfriend or girlfriend, that's chill. If you like to get nasty AF with someone you haven't even met in person, that's fine (as long as they are down for that, too).

It's a good place to get graphic because sexting is visual. The whole brain-game thing applies here. You can think of sexting as a virtual striptease. This was my best lesson from that dirty-talk workshop. The instructor explained that we should start by just describing what we were wearing, even if it wasn't something we were actually wearing. Try to describe everything in intimate detail. You want the other person to be able to imagine exactly what you're imagining.

Personally, I like to get right to the dicks, but everyone is different.

THREE TYPES OF SEXTERS

Obviously, everyone is different and special and unique as a unicorn, but I've distilled sexters into three main archetypes. This is based off both workshops I've taken and taught, as well as a lot of experience. I've written more sexts for my friends than I can possibly count. You're welcome, my friends' partners.

Not everyone is into everything I'm into, it turns out. My friend Lauren once asked me to help her craft a sext to a guy she was casually seeing. He had sent her something dirty, and she wanted to respond with equal steaminess. Yes, people do sometimes ask for third-party advice on sexting, and it's okay to do this if your source is trusted (Hi, it's me, Gigi!) and you don't tell the person whom you're sexting (unless it's a partner because obviously the source knows that person).

We were on our way to a bar after work. I took Lauren's phone. I couldn't exactly dictate a text to her on a crowded New York City street (though it is New York and weirder things have happened; I once saw a person simultaneously shitting himself and jerking off on the C Train).

I texted Lauren while writing this book to see if she had a copy of the infamous sext. She doesn't have it anymore, but she told me she wishes she did because it was so good. (Then why didn't you sext it, Lauren, huh???) I remember it being something like, "I want you to fill me with your rock-hard cock and spurt hot come all over me." Or something like that. Totally not even that bad, right?

Right? Anyone? Hello?

Whatever, guys. She took the phone back, read the text, looked at me, and read the text again. "Um. No way. I cannot send this." She deleted it. I was a little bit offended, but it wasn't my text to send, and we had a lot of wine to drink at this happy hour, so it was time to go.

Occasions like this helped me maneuver and categorize people into groups of sexting behaviors. Other teachers have created similar groups, I'm sure, but the ones I came up with were quite anthropological, if I do say so myself.

Gigi, shut the fuck up and tell me which kind of sexter I am.

Romantic

You might be asking, *How the hell can someone send a sext that's romantic?* Sexting is limitless, and what qualifies as sexting varies from person to person. Sometimes, sexting isn't about discussing clitorises and nutsacks but more about sensual language. Romantic sexters prefer beautiful language inspired by poetry. You know, softcore-style.

They like the more Shakespearean sexiness than Pornhub-level raunchiness. I don't necessarily mean, "Thou hast such delicate hands," or "Thou art a hot piece of delightfully plump booty." It can totally be about sex. Maybe instead of focusing on someone's penis or vulva, you pull the focus to other erogenous zones like the neck or back.

You're not lame if this is the kind of sexting you like. Fuck anyone who makes fun of you for wanting to write sweet romance sexts over dirty sexts. You do you.

Examples of romance sexts:

Your lips are so luscious and soft. I want to taste them.
*I wish I could put my hand on the small of your back and slide it down.**

---

* I am not good at this kind of sexting, clearly.

Cheeky

I love the word *cheeky*. It's got that pinup-girl feel. I think we should bring that word back to style. A cheeky sexter is someone who talks about all the dick, vag, and titty-fucking stuff without going so overboard you need a napkin to wipe your seat up after reading it. If your style is cheeky, you're getting into the dirtier stuff. You use curse words and talk directly about sex.

These sexts are usually more direct and straightforward. There are not a ton of adjectives or adverbs. It's just a sexy, straight-up description or demand. I'd say most people are cheeky sexters. It's a hybrid between being romantic and being filthy as fuck.

Examples of cheeky sexts:

I want to fuck you right now.
I wish your cock were in my mouth.
I'm so wet right now.

Filthy

Clearly, I'm a filthy fucking bitch when it comes to sexting. These are those sexts that are so wildly descriptive and visceral, you feel like you've been fucked after reading it. I'm talking down-and-dirty, balls-to-the-wall, taking-no-prisoners messages of explicit lust.

Anyone can become a filthy sexter. It just takes some imagination and a little faith. Just kidding. You just need adjectives. Rule #2 of sexting: The more adjectives, the dirtier the sext.

Examples of filthy sexts:

*I want you to sit on my face and soak my lips with your hot pussy
    juice.*
*Will you put your fat, thick cock inside me and pinch my nipples till I
    scream and fuck me until I come?*

Phew. KK. Moving on.

None of these archetypes are static. No need to suddenly feel
pressured like, "Fuck. Which sexter am I? I wrote that one sext
with two adjectives and one time I talked about a girl's forearms.
Who am I??"

You don't just fall into one box and call it a day. People can fluc-
tuate from category to category based on mood or level of comfort.
Sometimes a sext can be cheekier because you were in a meeting and didn't have time to write *pink, wet, slippery, juicy* in every
single message. You're a busy lady. Perhaps you just started dating
someone and don't want to talk about a cock/clit/taint yet. That is
completely fine.

HOW TO BE A DOPE SEXTER

Have you found yourself or are you currently finding yourself
agonizing over a sext? We've all been there, boo. If you're wondering how to take a sext to the next level, just add more descriptive
words. If you think something might be too explicit, take a few
words out. Keep it simple. Or not, you know? Sometimes you just
fucking go for it and hope for the best. In general, the more detail
with which you describe a sexual thing you want your partner to
do to you, or vice versa, the better. It's like creative writing. You

want the other person to be transported into your sexy fantasy for a hot minute.

The only thing that helps with the anxiety of sexy texting is doing it over and over again. Even then, it's still nerve-racking the first time you engage with a new partner.

I managed to hone my sexting skills because of this tax lawyer I was semi-dating, semi-fucking in my early twenties. He had the most boring job in the entire world and therefore had the most incredible imagination. He pushed me out of my comfort zone every single time he messaged me. We would send each other dirty, filthy sexts all day, every day whenever he was due to come to New York on business. I was constantly forced to reinvent what I thought was sexy and come up with new and interesting ways to turn him on. By the sheer volume of sexts, I became an expert. That's all it takes, regular practice. Rule #3: The more you sext, the better you get.

You have to remind yourself that you are a boss-ass bitch. It takes a confident woman to go for it with a sext. So what if it doesn't go as planned? So some person doesn't like that you mentioned wanting to get double penetrated bent over the living room couch. Fuck it. On to the next thing. You are the shit, and if someone doesn't love your sext, whatever. You learn from that experience and move on. Someone else will probably be into that in the future. Are you actually going to date someone who makes you feel shitty over something as stupid as a text message? Really?

As Mal Harrison, the director of the Center for Erotic Intelligence and brainchild of the sex column *Ms. M*, always says, the only thing normal about human sexuality is its variety. Don't let someone who shames you for trying something outside the box bring you down.

Try weird shit. I know it's scary and awkward, but you just have to do it. Think about your greatest fantasies and write them down in your phone notes. Send them in pieces to whomever you're sexting. Be creative with your sexts.

Listen to your partner and take notes. Sexting is trial and error. You have to test things out and see what works. It's highly likely some of the shit you say won't land the way you want it to. Just remember, this happens to everyone. I've had plenty of sexts that ended in silence. I've said some seriously fucked-up shit. I once told a guy I wanted to anally fist him. That didn't work out for me. I took a risk. I didn't even want to actually anally fist him. I had seen a porn vid with anal fisting and wanted to say it in a sext. Fuck it.

Now, I did learn from that experience. *Mental note: If I'm going to talk about anally fisting someone, perhaps I should figure out if they're interested in anal stuff to begin with. Are they into having things up their asses?*

Each person you're sexting has different preferences for what turns them on. If you talk about a gang bang fantasy and your partner doesn't seem to be into it or changes the subject, just take note of that and don't talk about gang bangs next time.

Rule #4: Ask yourself, *Would I want this sext?* Before you send a sext, any sext, ask yourself if you'd want to see this message sent from another person. This will help you gauge whether or not this is a good message to send. Case in point, I wouldn't want someone to sext me about anally fisting me. I should have run that one through my internal barometer before typing it out willy-nilly and shooting it into the world.

When you're sexting, there is a lot of ego involved. It feels like shit to have someone tell you that what you sent is inappropriate or uncomfortable, either directly or with silence. It's easy to simply wrap yourself up inside your own head and vow to never sext that person again. This is silly and won't serve you. Be willing to take the feedback and move on with your life.

WHEN SHOULD YOU SEND A SEXT?

The ultimate question. I often ask myself when I should be sending sexy text messages. I have an in-box full of questioning readers wondering when they should or should not send a sext. I have many friends and students who want to know if it's ever inappropriate or ill-timed to hit someone up with a description of their pussy. As they say, timing is everything.

There is no definitive answer. Hence the questions and bewilderment. It really depends on your relationship with the person you're sexting. If you're with someone you trust, you can likely just got for it. Actually, you can pretty much always go for it with whomever it is you're seeing. If you send a sexy text and they affirm the text with a sexy response, you're in the clear.

Timing isn't everything with sexts of the text-only variety. When I say *text-only,* I mean no photos or videos. Obviously, a picture of your titties is a wonderful thing to receive, just maybe not when your partner is sitting at his or her desk with coworkers aplenty sitting around him.

My favorite time is when you're waiting for your partner to get home from a long day at the office. A thing I once sent an ex-boyfriend: *When you get home, I'm going to kiss you so much. I am going to stick my tongue down your throat until you choke, but in a cute way*

☺." Just yesterday I sent my husband a text that said, *"As soon as I see you, I'm going to suck your cock. I miss your cock!"* Other times I straight up just send pictures of my tits for effect. The little things, you know?

If you know your partner is having a rough day, a hot text message can help lift their mood. Remind your partner you're at home waiting to get down and dirty. It can boost your confidence to be reminded that you're a hot piece of ass. Pretty much anytime you're feeling a little frisky, you can send a sext. Just remember to look out for the other person's response and tailor your messages accordingly. If they aren't into it, stop sending sexts to them.

Rule #5: Don't sext them at work over GChat before asking what they are currently doing in that moment. If you're going to send a sext, keep it relegated to a person's phone. If a person has their screen open and you send a dirty message, you risk getting them in trouble or, at the very least, embarrassing them in front of coworkers. I once had a friend who was screen sharing during a presentation have a raunchy-ass GChat pop up from her boyfriend. Her coworkers teased her about it for weeks. She's awesome and was able to brush it off and not give a fuck, but this isn't the case for everyone. If it's going to ping on a screen other than their mobile, don't sext while they're at work.

In sum, pretty much anytime is a good time for sexting as long as you know only their eyes will see said text message. My exes have opened their Snapchats during meetings and seen pictures of my tits. I wish I could say this has only happened once. It hasn't. Has this happened with my husband? I just asked him and he said, "Ummmm . . . yes. I actually had to change the preview option on my phone so it doesn't show your messages because they're so raunchy and I get so many of them." What can I say? He's fine with it.

WHAT DO I EVEN SAY?

Getting the conversation going is the hardest thing next to lulls. You're not the only one sitting around for hours trying to think of something sexy-but-not-creepy-but-hot. If you want to set the mood, try some sexual openers. As a general rule, something in the cheeky category is usually the way to go. (Just hope the person on the receiving end isn't like my most recent ex. He liked to send me thumbs-up emoticons when I sexted him, and I am still traumatized. Thank god my husband knows how to get into it. Blessings.)

All that being said, saying "go for something cheeky" is all fine and well, but that still leaves you wondering what the F to say. *Where are my concrete examples, bitch?* Chill the fuck out. Here are some ideas for openers:

What are you wearing?
I wish you were here right now. I'm so horny.
I'm so wet.
I had a dream you were fucking me last night.
I want to fuck as soon as you get here.
I want you.
I can't stop thinking about you naked.
I liked those pants you were wearing yesterday. Do they come off easily?

You know, nothing too intense (no visual descriptors of dicks and/or labia) but straightforward and to the point. If you sext someone one of the above lines and you get either silence, a subject change, or an awkward response—drop it and move on to either another conversation (or another person. Your call).

HOW TO GET A SEXT, GOOD OR BAD

Hot take: It's just as important to be good at *getting* a sext as it is to be good at *sending* one. We never emphasize the feelings of the person getting a sext. We always focus on the sender. If you get a sext (whether unsolicited, weird, or hot), you have to shuffle through your own emotions to figure out how to respond (or not respond).

Getting a weird or awkward sext is enough to make anyone want to slowly die inside. As usual, you're not alone. Getting a tragic sext is basically a rite of passage to becoming a woman.

One time, I was setting up a date with a Tinder dude, when out of nowhere he sent me something about going back to his apartment to take a bath together (romantic-style text). I hadn't even met this person before. I was not into it. Perhaps some women would be interested in that kind of message. I was not here for it. Should you get a sext that makes you want to slice your skin off with a disposable razor, and you want to tell a creepshow to fuck off, that is totally fine. You are your own woman and are entitled to do or say whatever the fuck you want.

But let's not play. Sometimes you get a sext that is fucked up from someone you were actually jibing with (or thought you were jibing with). Sometimes your long-term boyfriend or girlfriend can even say something that has nothing to do with anything you want ever. Like, *Where did this text about slipping a cucumber in my cunt come from, Melissa? Seriously.*

It's fine, even though it doesn't feel fine. It doesn't necessarily mean this person is sick in the head; they were probably just trying something on for size. The rules of sexting clearly state you should try weird shit. None of us know what the hell we're doing. If I had to lay a bet, I'd say that 98 percent of people who send a gross, weird sext do not think it's weird or gross. We're all just trying to get off. Sending a weird thing is not going to help someone in this quest. Now, obviously, there are "takers" out there who send something with the intention of making you feel disgusting (without your consent) because it gets them off, but these are outliers. In this case, this person is a taker because they are taking your peace of mind. They didn't send the "weird" thing to make you happy, they sent the weird thing to make them happy. See the difference?

If you get a bizarre sext, think about what you're going to do next. You're a confident woman. Let them know that wasn't something that turned you on or simply steer the conversation in another direction if you're not in the mood to spell it out. Clear communication is usually preferable, but these relationships are nuanced and diverse. This might be someone you're simply casually sexting as opposed to a serious partner. It's your call.

If this is someone you're casually dating and your lady-boner is totally killed by this thing you've been sent, you might want to take a look at the new relationship as a whole. If one sext could make you get over this budding romance, it probably wasn't meant to be. I'm all for giving second (or third) chances, but this is a red flag you should consider.

If it made you feel weird for a few minutes (or seconds) and then you were over it and are still into the person, move on. It's not that big of a deal.

THE BIG FOUR: THINGS TO REMEMBER WHEN YOU GET A SEXT (WHETHER GOOD OR BAD—BUT MOSTLY BAD, PROBABLY)

Empathy

Approach sexting with empathy rather than straight-up rejection or hostility. Instead of ignoring it or refuting their attempts to engage you, try being empathetic about where they're coming from.

I'm not, like, encouraging you to entertain a gross-ass person. Women are highly socialized to roll over and be nice to people who are awful. But this doesn't mean you should always default to being a fuckgirl.

If you're not into it and were never that into it, this was likely a nail in the coffin. Just remember that this is a human being with human feelings. Then, if you say it wasn't chill and they respond with some douchebag aggressive text, feel free to go off. You probably won't make them a better person, but they deserve to hear it.

Understanding

Figure out the motivations for this sext and try to make sense of it. Take a minute to process your feelings and consider how they might be feeling as well. This will dictate your response.

Context

Answer these questions: What is the context of this sext? Where are you? Where is the other person? Is this a new conversation? One you were already having?

The context of a sext is pretty important. If you were in the middle of a sexting conversation and he or she said something that was not okay, it might have been an error in judgment. If you're sitting at your desk at work, minding your own business, and suddenly get a random text about butt plugs from a guy or girl you just started seeing and it makes you feel icky, that's a different situation altogether. I think all my hetero and bisexual girls out there can vouch that we've all gotten a "Hey, how are you?" message on Tinder, followed by a picture of a raging boner.

Relationship

What is your relationship to the person sending this sext? Is it a casual thing? Is it your long-term boyfriend or girlfriend? How much do you like this person? This last question is the most important one of all. How into it are you? Lukewarm, super down, kind of meh, not into it at all?

But there is more to it than that. This whole jungle of sexting, texting, dating, and loving is fucking complicated and confusing. Sometimes you get a really good sext from someone you are super into, a hot sext from someone you're not into, a bad sext from someone you're into, a bad sext from someone you're not into. There is literally no limit to how fucked up this can be.

If you're wondering how to respond, just follow this magic tree.

WHEN YOU GET A HOT SEXT: How much you like this person versus how the sext made you feel.

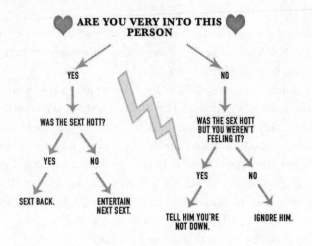

ARE YOU VERY INTO THIS PERSON

YES → WAS THE SEXT HOTT?
- YES → SEXT BACK.
- NO → ENTERTAIN NEXT SEXT.

NO → WAS THE SEX HOTT BUT YOU WEREN'T FEELING IT?
- YES → TELL HIM YOU'RE NOT DOWN.
- NO → IGNORE HIM.

WHEN YOU GET A BAD SEXT: How much you like this person versus how awkward the sext made you feel.

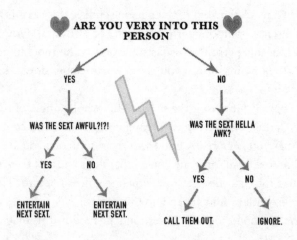

ARE YOU VERY INTO THIS PERSON

YES → WAS THE SEXT AWFUL?!?!
- YES → ENTERTAIN NEXT SEXT.
- NO → ENTERTAIN NEXT SEXT.

NO → WAS THE SEXT HELLA AWK?
- YES → CALL THEM OUT.
- NO → IGNORE.

Same chart, different feelings. If a sext is hot standing on its own, that's where you begin. You then apply context. Context is everything. If you got a sext that is objectively sexy, but it came from someone you're not into and do not want to fuck, it's going to be weird and make you feel gross or strange.

If you get a sext that is weird (to you) like, "I want to lick your feet heel to toe," but it came from someone you're really into, it can alter your feelings around it. (Unless you have a foot fetish, which is also totally kewl. We don't judge here.)

Now, you don't have to stick to the tree, boo. Nothing is ever binding. You are you own nasty woman, and you can do *whatever* you want. These are just mere suggests to help you out when you're in a bind and aren't sure how to proceed. Dating is such a pain in the ass.

A FEW RULES ON NUDE PHOTOS

Do not save your photos to the cloud or on your GDrive—or anywhere else where someone could get access to them. We should totally live in a world where you don't need to worry about people using nude photos against you. We should be able to accept that everyone has a body and photos of that body naked. Alas, people may try to use nudes against you as blackmail or for revenge. We talked about harassment already in chapter 4. Using nude photos to exploit or hurt someone is a form of harassment and digital violence.

When in doubt, use a service with disappearing photos. I enjoy using Snapchat for porn pics of myself. As Cindy Gallop says, the founders will never admit this, but that's what it was created for: sending nude photos and sexting. Obviously, people can screenshot these photos. You'll get a notification and should never sext that person again, but they still have the photo. You can never truly eliminate risk.

Which brings me to the last rule. Don't take photos with your face or any identifiable tattoos or body parts present. Even if you love the person and "know they would never send anyone your pictures," you have to take precautions. People are fucking assholes. Never take body shots where your face is in the frame. If you have a tattoo up the right side of your body, take photos of the left side. If you have tattoos all over your body, you can still send nudes, obviously, but do keep in mind you're more likely to be identified. Then again, there is Photoshop and someone could plant a tattoo or face on some random person's body and say it was you.

The internet is such a wonderful and horrible place. Be as careful as possible. I hate everything.

SOME THOUGHTS ON DIRTY TALK FROM SOMEONE WHO DOES IT A FUCKTON

Now that you have the information you need to sext, you can try talking dirty. For some of us, sexting is easier since we have time to think through what we're going to say. As a writer, I enjoy having a few minutes to think through everything I compose. I want the mood to be just right. This is not how it goes down with dirty talk. It's like doing stand-up: I'm funny in written words, but if I were in front of an audience, I would be about as funny as that tax authority I dated when I hung out with him in real life (i.e., literally not at all funny).

The upsides of dirty talk: You can just skip the words and make noises half the time and it works perfectly. A few deep, throaty moans and a couple of strategic "Oh, yes! *Yes!*" and "OOooOOOOo" and you're in the gold, my friend.

Unpopular opinion: Smoke marijuana before sex stuff. If you are someone who enjoys a little weed, have some marijuana before you get down and dirty. It heightens all your senses, especially touch. It blasts me into another universe, and suddenly I'm chattering away like I'm in my own, feminist adult movie. It feels a little dreamy and ups my confidence. I'm also so horny at that point that it doesn't even matter.

A good thing to remember is that this person you're doing the sex things with is into you already, hence why they are here naked, doing the sex things. You can say things (or not say things) and the likeliness that they will still fuck you is pretty high.

AD-LIB TIME, BITCH—YOU KNOW YOU'RE READY

And just when you thought this chapter could not be more fun, here are some exercises to sharpen your skills and your tongue. Welcome back to seventh grade, y'all. We are going to do some ad-lib shit now.

We're all sexy, nasty women, and so we should use our words to show how kick-ass we are. Even if you're a wordsmith, sometimes you're like, *Fuck. How many ways can I tell someone to stick their cock in me? I cannot think of a single original way to tell my girlfriend to tie me to the bed and spank me. I am fresh out of material up in this bitch.*

There are a few different kinds of ad-libbing approaches you can choose from, depending on the feel you're going for. Are you being a sexy dominatrix tonight? Are you trying to get your partner in the mood to take control? Are you feeling submissive? Are you just trying to get shit going right now? Your words have a lot of control and a lot of power. They can drive a sexual experience any way you'd like. Sex is just as much auditory as it is touch, taste, and smell. Make the most of it.

Ad-Libbing, Round 1: The Compliment
Option 1:
> I love it when you (verb) my (adjective) (noun).

Option 2:
> You have the most fantastic (adjective) (noun).

Option 3:
> You're so good at (verb+ing) my (noun).

Ad-Libbing, Round 2: The Suspense
Option 1:
> I'm going to (fill in the blank).

Option 2:
> I really want to (verb) your (noun) later.

Option 3:
> If you're not good, I'm going to (fill in the blank).

Ad-Libbing, Round 3: The Request
Option 1:
> I want (fill in the blank).

Option 2:
> Will you (verb) your/my (noun) on/in your/my (noun)?

Option 3:
> I've been naughty. You should (fill in the blank).

Ad-Libbing, Round 4: The Demand
Option 1:
Put your (noun) inside/on/in of my (noun).
Option 2:
Take your (blank), and touch my (adjective) (noun).
Option 3:
(verb) all over my (adjective) (noun) until I (verb).

ANOTHER FUN EXERCISE: HAND THE PHONE OVER

Have one of your trusted friends craft a sext for you. Sometimes you just legit need someone to take the reins and handle the situation for you.

Why? Your friend loves you and wants you to get some ass. They also have no skin in the game other than your happiness. They know what to say and aren't going to get caught up in a flurry of emotions and anxiety about the other person not being into it. We have the power to be our own worst enemy. We don't send what we want to send, or we freak out over sending what we wanted to send and end up screwing ourselves (and definitely not in a good way).

Giving your phone to a friend relieves you of the stress and puts the challenge in their hands. Be sure this is a friend you really, truly trust. This is not some shenanigans to get into with Josie from your tennis team, whom you've known for two months. It also works much more smoothly if your friend also has someone you can sext for her (or him, or them).

Again, this exercise isn't for everyone. It's merely a suggestion.

It's possible that watching the ease with which someone sexts can give you the confidence to handle it yourself.

FEEDBACK IS ALWAYS IMPORTANT
SO, GET IT TOGETHER

Feedback during sexting and dirty talk is important and should be done regularly. A badass bitch like you does not need to put up with shit she's not into. Ever. You give different kinds and levels of feedback for different relationships. If you're with someone long term, it might be easier for you to be like, *Stop that now!* if they are doing something weird and not sexy. If you don't know the person that well, you may just not chill with them anymore if they get creepy on you. The important thing is listening and communication. Be open to giving and receiving concrete suggestions. Now, it's easier said than done when it comes to feedback. I can tell you to be honest and open until my clit turns blue, but we both know that isn't going to work.

So how do you give honest feedback without turning into my friend the silent jellyfish?

Giving feedback to a new partner is a nerve-racking task. The truth is, if you don't want to downright say, "That was a gross thing to say," you don't have to. You are the leader of your own actions. If you want the person you're seeing to know that was a fucking vile thing to say, opt for, "I prefer X over gang bangs," or "I'd much rather you tie me up and spank me." Shift the focus. It is so easy to shift the focus over text. Sexting is weird AF, and your partner is not going to repeat something again if he or she didn't get a pro-verbial standing ovation. If you outline exact scenes you're into, in all likeliness, your new boyfriend or girlfriend (or Tinder date or whatever) will follow suit. Take their ability to listen, absorb, and learn as a sign of whether they'd be a genuine person to consider for the long term (if that's what you're looking for).

If you're in a relationship with someone, this endeavor is, by and large, easier. You trust this person. At least you should. If your relationship is healthy and equal, you can tell him or her that something they sexted you was a little awkward. Obviously, no one wants to bruise an ego—male, female, or otherwise. Sexting is already ballsy. Having the gumption to pick up the phone in the first place and graphically describe your pussy and the objects you'd like to put inside of it is bold, and I commend your fine ass for doing that and your partner's fine ass for coming through.

If you don't want to come right out and say, "I didn't really like that you sexted me thirteen times today about lubing up your fist and gently shoving it up my asshole," you also have the power to shift the conversation away from that sort of sext. There is no need to text all your friends and let them know your partner might be into gang bangs and you're really concerned. Chill.

Instead of going along with it, offer some radio silence and see if that takes care of it. If not, just sext something completely different. Shift away from anal fisting (if you're not into anal fisting) and move into sitting on your partner's face, stroking her clit, or playing with his balls. Nuance is perfectly acceptable if that's the route you feel comfortable with. Remember the Big Four main things to remember during sexting? #2 is *understanding*. Your partner is not trying to make you feel gross. Eight out of ten times, he or she probably doesn't even want to actually fist your anus. Sexting is a fantasy. It's a place to test out the waters, after all. If you're not showing any interest in it, your partner will get the memo (as if anyone sent memos anymore, though, seriously).

In that same vein, pay attention to how your partner is responding to your sexts. If you get graphic and begin describing a scene and aren't being met with enthusiasm, shift gears. There is nothing wrong with your fantasy, and there is nothing wrong with your partner's fantasy. Sexual preferences are as varied as an earring collection. There is no wrong or right way. You both want to make each other happy and hard/wet.

If you listen, you can improve your sexting game and learn new shit along the way. Sexting helps build your confidence as a nasty woman. Believe it or not, bb, you will get closer to finding love if you start to gain self-worth through your own sexuality. Once you become a woman who sexts and talks dirty with assertiveness, you start to feel that way about yourself in your bones. You begin to understand your own sexual power and abilities to turn someone on.

Now that you have the tools to finesse your sex connection and keep things hot in a relash and a casual thang, the next step is getting things a little . . . kinked.

How to Be a Kinky, Sexy Bitch

When you're a nasty woman, looking to explore new avenues of hot-ass sex is only natural. I'm with you, girl.

Kinky sex is the center of so many fantasies but something so few of us know how to ask for (or pull off). How do you ask your sex partner to casually choke you out or tie you to a bed without sounding insane? Do you buy some handcuffs and swing them around, dancing to Beyoncé until your boo gets the picture? Do you just bend over and screech, *"Pour hot wax on my ass cheeks, babe!"*? A healthy mix of the two approaches? Something else entirely?

If you're going to slay in life, you should slay in bed. Let's talk about all that *Fifty Shades* shit in a way that doesn't make me want to projectile-vomit all over myself. (Sorry, E. L. James, but you know you fucked us up, but also can I have some of your money? Maybe? No? Maybe?) Right up in here is the skinny on everything from role play to BDSM to pegging. Kinky sex is something so many of us crave but are afraid to make happen. With all due respect, fuck that.

I talked to nearly all the people I know in the kink community for this chapter. I hit up everyone from Tina Horn of the *Why Are People Into That?!* podcast, to Carol Queen, the resident sexologist/badass bitch of the feminist sex toy store Pleasure Chest, to

Sandra LaMorgese, a dominatrix with a Ph.D.—and many others who helped me fine-tune and comprehensively pinpoint the important shit you need to know about kink.

I consider myself relatively kinky, but I don't know how to do a lot of things. For instance, I'm unsure of how to safely tie knots because I am incompetent (seriously, I still use the two-bunny-ears trick to tie my shoes), nor do I know how to nail a scrotum to a wall because I have shaky hands (LOL forever. This is probably the least rational reason for why I should never attempt to slice a nail through a ball sack, but whatever).* We're actually not going to get *that* into ball-sack nailing because none of you newbies should be trying that anyway.

Here is everything you need to know about getting kinky—how to have those initial conversations, what a wee bit of BDSM can do for your health, and how to get started.

Come into my dungeon. Just kidding. I don't have a dungeon. And not all kink is even performed inside of a dungeon. Probably not even the majority of it.

FIRST THINGS FIRST: WHAT IS KINK?

Stephen James Buford, founder of *Raw Attraction Magazine,* told me in an email that the thing people get wrong most often about kink and BDSM is believing the misconception "that it is only for strange people and that you must be slightly insane to do it."

---

* Also, I didn't know that was even something people do until Sandra dropped it into casual conversation like it was no big deal. I, of course, pretended it was 100 percent no big deal so she wouldn't think I was a loser. I have a complex, clearly.

Kink may sound like some wild, scary thing people only do in fringe groups of the underworld, but that's actually not true at all. According to a 2005 survey from Durex, 36 percent of adults have used blindfolds, handcuffs, or other forms of basic restraints and sensory deprivation during sexual play. This was a full six years before *Fifty Shades* popped up on the scene. According to a 2015 survey from MarieClaire.com, 85 percent of adults in America report trying some form of bondage. In short, people are into it.

So what is kink, exactly, and what does it include or not include? This is actually a more complicated question than you might think. Kink is an unconventional sexual behavior or combination of sexual behaviors. Anything outside of the regular, run-of-the-mill sexual practices you're used to could be considered kinky. Kinks range from the mild to the super dirty and "weird." People often think that kink has to be painful or in a dungeon. This is not true.

Dr. Emily Morse, a prolific sexologist and voice behind the *Sex with Emily* podcast, really puts it perfectly: Kink is whatever is outside of your comfort zone, whatever that comfort zone may be. Kink varies and differs from person to person. Handcuffs could be super kinky to you. A massage might be something you consider kinky.

Kink is a broad term that is hard to define. Lots of people have different ideas of what is kinky. Some people might be having kinky sex that isn't kinky because they don't consider it kinky. It's basically everything that is sexually atypical or outside of the "normal." Which is already fucked up because who gets to define what is "normal," anyway?

In the community, there is vanilla sex (sex that is not kinky), and there is kink. Again, whatever you consider one or the other is up to you. Yeah, I've got some feelings about this. Let me live.

Here is where it gets a little wishy-washy and confusing. Even I

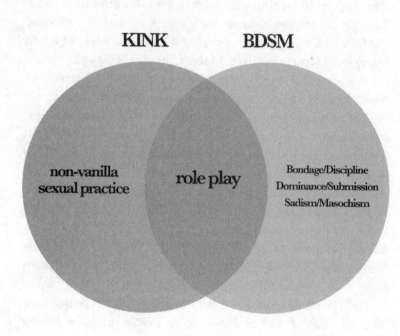

get confused. So I have a Venn diagram (see facing page) to try to explain this visually. BDSM is kink, but not all kink is BDSM—but it can be used interchangeably if you want to use it interchangeably (lots of people do this). It's about what makes you comfortable. Role play is kinky, but not all kink involves role play. Some role play is a part of BDSM. See? It's confusing. If I had to wager a guess, I'd have to say this comes from people a) not talking about sex in any capacity, leaving all of us to try to blindly figure out what the fuck is going on, and b) for whom sexuality is fluid and sex practices are nonrestrictive, therefore making them hard to define.

Someone might think dressing up as a nurse and giving their partner an enema is vanilla. I would call that kinky, but it's not my place to inform them about their own sex lives. That's their business.

Dr. Dulcinea Pitagora, sex therapist and founder of the show *KinkDoctor,* says that any sexual thing done between consensual partners, in a healthy way, is perfectly acceptable. Just because it seems odd to someone, why should it be up to them to judge you? We humans love anything taboo or naughty, and that's where kink gets its mojo. Kinky sex practices have become pretty mainstream, and more and more people are into trying them. When you've tried a lot of different things sexually, moving into some kink can be a great way to spice things up in a relationship or in your sex life in general.

Sandra LaMorgese, a dominatrix and Ph.D., subscribes to the role-play aspect of kink. Kink is more a fantasy. It's something you want to try or something you want to explore with a partner or otherwise. If you're kinky, it covers lots of things and trying different things.

You might also wonder what the difference is between a kink and a fetish. Like, is there a difference? Is this one and the same? Is that foot thing I like wherein a toe goes up my butthole a kink or what? It's nothing to be embarrassed about. It's confusing AF. A kink is an idea of something you want to try or something you enjoy doing—something you add on to playtime, but it is not consuming, whereas fetish is a part of you. A fetish is forever. It's a part of your system. It never goes away.

KINK IS IN YOUR CONTROL

Trying kink is totally in your control. I cannot emphasize this enough. What scares people shitless about bondage is the idea that they are going to submit to something they aren't comfortable with and wind up flipping out or dying.

Just because you are a sexually empowered woman does not mean you have to be down for weird sex stuff whenever (or at all, boo). If this is something you want to try, that's fantastic. It is a choice. It doesn't mean you have to do kink all the time. Your sex life does not have to transform into a dom-sub situation à la Christian and Ana if that isn't what you want. You can do some kink here and there, you can do it all the time, or you can do it not at all.

Consent is key. If you want to try kink, it in no way implies that consent goes out the window. Sandra says that consent is just as important as it is during vanilla sex practices. Consent is a big part of kink because when you're taking on different roles and trying new, potentially dangerous things, you can't not talk about it. One of the things that makes BDSM and kink so magical is the power you willingly give away or take. It lets you be in the moment and be very present.

The choice and consent aspects of kink are foundational to its success. When I was in my early twenties, I was casually hooking up with a guy I thought I trusted. Looking back, I clearly didn't know him that well and didn't trust him that much. He also had no idea what he was doing, but I was a child and didn't know that. For all his big talk about getting kinky, he was a novice at best.

I had never done bondage before, not even light choking. This man was quite a bit older than I, and I wanted to come across as very sexy and worldly. You know, super rad and down for anything. I decided to just dive in with a reckless abandon to maintain my cool-girl aesthetic.

In the span of about four minutes, I was tied up and ball-gagged, feet and wrists tied to each corner of the bed. The ball gag was sickly sweet; a jawbreaker meant to make it more fun, I guess? It hurt my teeth and mouth, stretching the corners of my cheeks uncomfortably. I was blindfolded. I couldn't tell him if this was okay or if it wasn't okay. I felt claustrophobic and afraid. I had a panic attack. I started screaming as much as I could and was shaking uncontrollably. He untied me. He was clearly shaken. We popped some champagne, watched *Modern Family,* and then had regular vanilla sex later.

This is a tale of caution. I wanted to be impressive so badly that I compromised my comfort and safety. This is not how you want your experiences with kink to be. I'm not entirely sure how much BDSM experience this guy had with kink or if he had decided to stock up on a ton of expensive gear on a whim. Regardless, as the dominant in this situation, he had a responsibility to make sure I was feeling safe and comfortable. He wasn't thinking about this during the sexual play. I'm no mind reader, but I don't believe he'd even considered it. Don't play dom-sub games with random people who don't know what they're doing. You might end up in a shit-your-pants-scary situation like I did. The dom has responsibility to the sub. Always.

I don't want this tale of woe to stop you from trying kink. Quite the contrary. I want to set you on a path of well-informed experiences that don't end in heart palpitations. As far as bad first times go, mine was tame. No lasting harm was done. But it's important to know that when you don't know what you're doing and don't trust the person you're doing those things with, it can go awry.

Remember that you are exploring these things for your own pleasure. You do not need to do kink to fit into some lens of what makes a sexy partner. Do not do anything that you do not want to do. You're not less sexy or cool or dope if you don't want to be tied up and gagged. If you're going to try kink, do it for yourself, not to please someone else. It's great to open yourself up to something your partner wants to try, but only if you feel safe doing it. You are your own fantasy, okay, boo?

BDSM: A NASTY WOMAN'S GUIDE

You hear a lot about BDSM but, like, do you really know what it even is? Not many people do, so it's fine. *BDSM* stands for *bondage, dominance, submission, masochism.* (It also includes *discipline, sadism,* and sometimes the *S* and *M* are referred to as *sadomasochism.*)

When I asked Dr. Kristie Overstreet, a clinical sexologist and psychotherapist, about BDSM, she really summed up how disorienting the understanding can be in a nutshell: "BDSM is consensual sexual expression, and it is not abuse. If you see a BDSM scene that involves knife or blood play, you may have a strong reaction to it, because it is outside of your comfort level. However, the participants in the scene consented and discussed the rules of the scene beforehand. Just because you may think it is abuse doesn't mean that it is."

BDSM comes in many shapes and sizes. On its surface, it may well look like abuse. Many scenes involve a person tied up, ruthlessly spanked or beaten, and yes, it can involve blood sometimes. The difference is the consent and understanding. All the people engaging have discussed their boundaries, how they want the scene to take place, and what they are and are not comfortable doing. They are doing this for their own pleasure, not because another person(s) forced them to take part. It is not coerced behavior in any way.

I'd love to delve into the intricacies of BDSM, shame, and lust, but I have to break down the basics. We can't possibly cover everything about how society feels about BDSM in one chapter. So we can only munch on the bones. The majority of people don't want to engage in sex like this (or, at least, don't admit it). Society is scared of BDSM. It bolsters the power of sexual freedom. It openly promotes and advocates for the human desire to give up or take control. That's some scary shit. So we censor it, and therefore, we can't talk about it. Our culture doesn't know how to talk about sex at all, let alone bondage and whether or not you're a sub, dom, or switch.

The different roles in BDSM are not finite and cast a rather wide net. There are subcategories that I'm choosing to omit and instead am choosing to focus on the most popular roles.

Here are some basic definitions to help you understand BDSM outside of the bullshit you find on the internet.

Different Roles

Dominant

A dom is the person with the control (not to be confused with taking away consent: every person in a scene, regardless of role, has power and control). The scene is a journey you lead as a dominant. It is the game, the fantasy. It describes everything that goes down both mentally and physically in the space. The "play" is the actions themselves. A dom might set a scene wherein the sub is a helpless kitten tied to the bed. The play is the actual tying to the bed and whatever else the dom does during the scene. Doms are the one who create the scene for both his or herself and the submissive. Both parties have power, but the dom exercises his or her will over the submissive, consensually. The dom takes pleasure in guiding the sub to new heights of pleasure and awareness. If there is a spanking given out, the dom gives the spanking. If there is bondage, the dom is the one doing the tying.

Subsets: Masters/Mistresses; Femdom

A master or mistress is a dom who is worshipped by the sub as a sort of overlord figure. A dom may choose to be a dominant but not want to be considered a master or mistress. It depends on what you want out of the scene.

A femdom is a female dominant. A femdom can also be a mistress or vice versa. This term is more of a way to categorize women in the scene, as the patriarchal culture in which we live finds it difficult to accept women in places of power over men. A femdom uses her particular female characteristics as a way to control and humiliate male or female clients. An example? Stepping on a cis-man's junk in stilettos.

Submissive

A submissive gives up control to the dom. A sub derives pleasure by giving up control and fully submitting to their dom. It turns a sub on to be dominated, enslaved, and/or consensually ravished. As a sub, you are still very much in control. You have set your boundaries and preferences up beforehand. The pleasure derived from the scene is as much about you as it is about the dom. If there is spanking to be given out, the sub is spanked. If there is bondage, the sub is the one tied up.

The raw power of being a submissive was beautifully described in the following story from Stephen James Buford:

> I am a heterosexual man but there was one BDSM scene that I was in where there were two other guys and two women. Towards the end of the scene the guys took me, stripped me na-ked, blindfolded me, put a rope mankini on me and beat me in front of about forty other people. I never particularly liked be-ing naked in front of other people, let alone beaten by two guys. It wasn't a sexual experience for me but it was a lesson in deep surrender. I couldn't do anything. There was deep love involved, especially when it finished. The four people in my scene came and hugged me for at least ten minutes. I had learned that it was OK to go to this level of surrender and submission in my life, there was no shame in it.

Subsets: Slave; Pet; Brat

A slave is a submissive who is at the complete mercy of the dom. You are quite literally a slave. Your dominant/master/mistress may make you lick his or her feet or clean his or her apartment or dungeon. Again, this is an interchangeable and fluid term.

Pets are submissives that aim to please the dominant in any way they can, much like a dog does its master. If you're a good pet, you get rewarded. If you're bad or don't take an order, you get punished. It is a way to dehumanize the sub for their sexual pleasure.

A brat is a submissive that gets off by being disobedient and getting punished as a result. The turn-on for the brat is not listening to the dom or resisting their control. Every time a brat is naughty, they might be met with spanking, caning, or some other form of punishment.

Switch

A switch plays both dominant and submissive roles or top/bottom roles. You may be a switch who leans dominant or submissive. You may fall right in the middle. Who you are in a scene may depend on the person you're engaging with. Perhaps with one partner you are a dom, but with another you fall into a submissive role. You may enjoy switching from a dom to a sub mid-scene. There is truly no limit to how these roles can be played.

BDSM is a healthy form of sexual expression. Sandra LaMorgese says it's healthy to express that part of yourself because suppression will destroy you. If you stay locked up inside of your own desire and never release it, you'll lose your mind.

Are you afraid of pain or of giving pain? Honestly, it's not even about that in the broader scheme of things. BDSM is less about pain and more about power dynamics and control. It isn't about someone taking control over you to hurt you (or for you to take control over someone to hurt them); it's about exploring different dynamics within your sexual relationship. It finds its influence through energy swirling between the participants and power exchange.

Sandra tells me that most clients aren't even into pain. During a session, she had a client just look at her feet for twenty-five minutes, and he was hypnotized. It was magical for him. BDSM shares qualities with hypnosis. It often allows a dom to bring a sub into the subspace* and then gently back out.

Kink is like yoga or a massage. It's a form of therapeutic release. Many do it as much for mental clarity and exploration as they do for sexual gratification.

It's not necessarily about the acts themselves but how the acts make you feel. Every single sex act you engage in should be consensual and enlightening. Nothing is ever out of your control. Everything should feel good, whatever it is you're trying. This practice is about being connected. You get high from dopamine and serotonin. If kink is something you're into, you turn on and get hyperaware. It's like jumping into a cold pool of water or doing a really intense kickboxing class. It's a high.

Sex therapist Dr. Pitagora explains that kink is about intense connection and the creation you get from your partner. It's about the whole experience. You are always in control of the situation,

---

* Subspace: An enlightened sense of being when engaging in bondage or kink. The sub goes into a trancelike state wherein they are totally free of the constraints of everyday life. You're in a zone, like an athlete. It's an energy dimension that is different from your normal reality. You're so high, you're away from the world—much like a pure state of meditation. It is an entirely new plane of existence. Subspace is experienced differently from person to person.

even if you're submissive. You have power, and consent is always present. It can change or stop at any time.

KINK AS THERAPY

Kink is used by some to explore past traumas. For some, it is a way to safely explore the skeletons in their pasts. This is not the reason everyone loves kink. Many, many kinksters engage in kink because they simply love the power dynamics and connections. Still, it is worth noting, kink, at its core, is not about fucking someone up; it's about healing and learning about your body. It is about experiencing your body and connecting to it.

I've heard many stories of women who experienced sexual abuse (or abuse in some form) who came to the BDSM community. Through its practices, they were able to confront the pain of their past, begin to heal, and get back in touch with their bodies to experience pleasure.

Kenna Cook, a sex educator and BDSM enthusiast, told the following story about her experience of reclamation and, ultimately, gaining true autonomy through kink.

I reclaimed my sexuality after an abusive marriage that was sex starved and emotionally destructive. When I first started dating again, I was afraid to have sex because of the shame I had received about expressing my desires for sex that looked different from heterosexual, missionary style. I started to explore porn and found myself drawn to folks that looked alternative. They were queerer than me, and their sex looked like it was full of pleasure.

I knew that I was a voyeur and I wanted to experience more of what looked like empowering sexuality for myself.

BDSM helped me learn to trust my partners through the negotiation and consent practices. I was scared the first time I asked someone to spank me. "What if I hated it? What if I liked it? What would they think of me?" All of my fears didn't have to stay inside my head because before-play negotiations, during play check-ins, and after-play aftercare made it so I was also in control and in communication with my partners about my experience. I wasn't silenced. I was finally allowed [to] exist.

I read a story of a girl who had been sexually abused as a child. She suffered from vaginismus as an adult as a result of her abuse. Her vagina tensed up and was impenetrable. Sex was excruciatingly painful. Once she came to the kink community, she was able to confront some of those past demons through the methods of control, pain, pleasure, and domination. It was a controlled space where she could look at her demons and stand against them. BDSM allowed her to take back much of the control she had lost as a child. It was her empowerment.

Feminista Jones, an activist and powerhouse, spoke powerfully about this topic in her own life when she played emcee at the Sex as Resistance conference, where I spoke in 2017.

Her story of overcoming past trauma to find lost sexual pleasure broke my heart and gave me hope. BDSM is not about pain, and it is not about torture; it is so much more than that. It can be a true coping mechanism. There are countless stories that present BDSM and role play as a way of working through the past. Lottie, a twenty-seven-year-old switch, offered the following thoughts on the giving and receiving of power and how it helped her cope with her own trauma:

> As a switch, I can move between both dominant and submissive roles. Dominance allows me to work through trauma by choosing to behave differently than my abuser did—it has helped me to realize that I can give intense experiences and have intense sex without it being psychologically or seriously physically harmful to anybody involved. Being totally in control of somebody else's experiences has helped me understand the feelings of power this gives, and I can enjoy that power without guilt. On the other hand, as a submissive, I enjoy completely giving over to my dom, and can enjoy sensations of pain, or rough sex, without feeling ashamed or afraid.

Sandra tells me that her clients use kink to cope in a truly granular way. Many of her clients relive the traumas with her, in a safe and controlled environment, to heal through role play. Re-enacting the memories that caused you harm is a way to heal for some. Whether it be a boss, a coworker who humiliated them, or a mother who was overbearing and smothering, the role play takes away the shame.

Carol Queen, the resident sexologist at Pleasure Chest, says that therapy in BDSM comes from the communication one experiences within the role-play context. It's not just therapeutic for those with a traumatic past but for those who have not had power or control in their lives.

Communication is so valorized and necessary that it becomes appealing to people with backgrounds where they may not have had communication at the forefront. You get to negotiate and have boundaries and be comfortable on your own terms. Consent and communication are critical components of all sex, regardless of type, but the particular focus in the BDSM community offers unmatched boundaries. People with traumatic backgrounds often don't feel like they have agency or control, and this type of play gives it back to them. It's a therapeutic space where you can say no. You can even say no right in the middle of something that's happening to you. You have the ability to be in total control. The BDSM community places emphasis on discussing one's boundaries. It is considered a vital, sexy element of the play. You don't always get there in other sexual situations (which is obviously super fucked up). With consent at the forefront, it makes it easier to communicate and set your boundaries. BDSM might feel violent in a superficial sense, but it is possibly the safest kind of sex there is. Don't get me wrong—all good sex should feel safe. The principles of open discussions in this community could teach more "traditional" sex-havers something.

Kink is about more than just therapy; it's just good for your overall health. Honestly, people are freaks. We're all weirdos. What holds us back from being weird is a fear of ostracization from our communities. A 2008 study from *The Journal of Sexual Medicine* found that people who engaged in kinky-sex practices were not at all depraved outliers of society. They were normal, regular people looking to enjoy a fruitful sex life with some whips, chains, and dildos. All people think about something that someone else might consider weird in the sheets. We just don't talk about it—which is fucked up and makes people think they are broken freaks who will never be loved.

I asked Sandra what it means to be truly sexually empowered. She told me that in order to achieve this state, you have to own who you are. Whatever it is, be true to it. Find out about yourself. Learn about your body. Find out who you are and then find a partner who's into that.

EVERYONE FINDS THEIR WAY TO KINK IN THEIR OWN WAY

There are myriad ways one finds their way to kink. Maybe you saw a super-sexy porn video where a group of women tied another hot woman to a Saint Sebastian's cross and you thought, *Oh, wow. I would like to be tied to a cross.* Maybe you've read erotic novels with BDSM at the center story line and wanted to try whipping someone. Perhaps you have a partner who is really into kink play. However you find your way there (if you do find your way there), it is all legitimate and wonderful. Sexual exploration is the tits. There is no limit to the ways you can play. We're all just a bunch of hot-ass perverts trying to come our faces off. Whether it be through spanking or a bunny-looking vibrator on our clitorises.

Tina Horn, a former professional dom and creator of the *Why Are People Into That?!* podcast says that she got kinky because her partner was into it. She didn't just spring from the womb in a spandex strap-on and a corset, ready for business. She came around to kink much like one comes around to a new type of cuisine. The key is to look at any kind of sexual play with a sense of curiosity rather than revulsion. Maybe you think it really is fucked up and want nothing to do with it. That's okay. It's not for everyone. But don't limit yourself because you're afraid of the unknown. That ain't cute.

Give yourself some room to explore. You may want to try being a dominant and find it's not for you. You may think you want to be a submissive or a slave and realize that's not for you. Be willing to explore these roles and adapt. If you don't like something, do not continue to do it. At the end of the day, it's about what makes you happy and fulfilled. I'm not saying kink will bring you fulfillment; I'm just offering it up as an option. Being a nasty, empowered-ass woman means exploring every sexual foray with a sense of self and agency. Sex is one of life's purest pleasures, and life is too fucking short to have sex in a way you don't want to, you know?

HOW TO BRING UP KINK (AND HOW TO GET STARTED)

You may be so turned on by all the above information (maybe the trauma stories not included, but I'm not one to judge) that you want to grab a riding crop and a blindfold and party on down to Kink Town.

But how do you get started with all those conversations, safe words, enthusiastic consent, and set boundaries? How do you tell your partner you want to do some out-of-the-box shit after he or she gets home from work tonight?

You could send them some photos of girls or boys tied up with ball gags, but that doesn't seem right. That might scare your boo. You can't just scream, "Tie me to the bed!" in the middle of sex. That might be confusing or even a little terrifying if you've never tried that before. It could work in some cases (I'm sure it has), but safety and empathy are always the chief concerns. You don't want to be like me, where you just throw yourself down on the bed when your partner has a bunch of bondage gear, either. That was

scary as shit. It took me a few years to go anywhere near bondage gear again. You never want to be the person responsible for
another person's trauma. Sex is about releasing inhibitions and getting down with your bad self, not walking away with nightmares
that last circa forever.

You have to talk everything through. I mean everything.
Dr. Pitagora says communication is integral to BDSM play of any
kind. You have to be very clear about this piece before you try
anything kinky. But Esther Perel, the world-renowned sex therapist, says in her book *Mating in Captivity* that talking is often the
antithesis of eroticism, that desire needs mystery to flourish. However, it's not what you talk about, it is how to talk about it. Talking
can be the antithesis of eroticism if you talk about sex in a boring,
structural way. Sitting down with a drawing board and outlining
exactly how a scene is going to play out doesn't inspire many an
engorged clitoris. You have to spark the conversation in a sexy, excited way. Think of it as a form of foreplay.

Auntie Gigi is going to be real with you. There is no magical
way to make a conversation about trying new sex stuff not weird.
This conversation is probably going to be pretty awkward. It's not
every day that you're like, "Hi, babycakes. Can you spank me with
a wooden spoon while I call you Daddy tonight? K, thanks, love
you, bye."

Honestly, you have to be willing to make it awkward. Fuck it.
This is an uncomfortable conversation, and it might be weird. You
have to be willing to say the wrong thing and feel weird about it.
Acknowledge that weirdness. "I want to have a conversation about
sex, but I know it's going to be weird," is a good place to begin.

There is no right or wrong way to start on your path toward
kink. It all begins with where your sexual interests are. Start with

your fantasies and see what comes out of that. Tap into yourself and focus on what turns you on. A little spanking? Some dirty talk? The thought of being gagged and bound? Pegging your partner with a twelve-inch purple dildo?

You have to go into these practices with a willingness to get to know yourself. Go to a sex shop, watch porn, and see what tickles your proverbial fancy. Listen to what makes your clit tingle. You know the feeling. It's like a big shot of electricity and a warm tug—go from there. Do some exploring and some research. Tina says to read as much as you can. Get every nonfiction sex book that's highly rated on Amazon and read that shit.

If you're finding it too difficult to just come right out and say what you want to explore with your partner, start by talking about fantasy and about fantasies you've had in the past.

Watch some porn. Try sharing a porn that involves some bondage. There is a ton of porn devoted to bondage.

If you're more comfortable with photographs, you could show your partner some erotic imagery. Try Googling *shibari*—the Japanese art of rope tying. There are some very gorgeous photos that could turn your partner on. Check out *The Seductive Art of Japanese Bondage* by Midori. Even the cover art will get you wet.*

You still don't have to jump into a kinky sex scene after watching a gang bang bondage porno just because it turned you on. Often making the step from exploring your desires to actually acting them out is a difficult transition for one or both (or multiple) partners.

---

* Like I said, I am super not able to tie knots, but that doesn't mean *shibari* imagery isn't hot as fuck. You don't have to try everything you see or experience every single thing that gets you going.

Baby steps. Move slowly. All people need to feel like they're safe and in control of the environment around them. Everyone needs to feel like their needs and wants are being tended to and appreciated. Come out slowly about your needs. Let your partner in on your desires. Let them take this journey with you.

When it comes to us ladies, we need to have more confidence around our sexuality in general. This hasn't been something we've been encouraged to do, by and large. The more open we can be in talking about our sexuality and what our desires are, the more comfortable we'll be in our own skin. What we need is permission to explore our desires without shame and repercussions.

Exploring both fantasy and kink is about learning about yourself. Figure out what you are about and who you are as a person. Then you can explore kink with full control and authority. You come out slowly, and the more comfortable you feel, the more you can reveal about your desires.

The key is opening the pathway to communication. Once the dialogue starts, you can steer it where you want it to go. Don't shut down the communication by saying no to everything.

Now, if you don't want to share everything with your partner, that's your decision. You don't have to make everything about the two of you. It's okay to have some fantasies that you want to keep and own for yourself. If you want to explore them with your partner, then reveal them slowly.

This goes both ways, the care and empathy. If your partner wants to try something you aren't into, you can always try something less intense and work up to it. Don't just shut your partner down. Keep the door open. Be open to possibilities. Vulnerability is true empowerment.

Make the conversation about you and your partner. Let your

partner know that he or she can tell you anything and you'll still be there. If your boo wants to wear a diaper during sex and you aren't down to try that, don't be a dick about it.

Intense kink flourishes when you practice it with someone you trust. Don't get adventurous with some random piece of shit you just met on Tinder or in line at Whole Foods or at the gym.

Also, do not go straight to dangerous shit the first time you try kink. I recommend starting with simple Velcro handcuffs and a T-shirt blindfold. You don't have to buy a ton of expensive gear. Find out if you love kink before you go forth and buy a $400 bespoke corset, hand-woven with roses and spikes. The sex swing can wait until you figure out if this is something you want to keep exploring. You're not less cool for not having eighty-three riding crops to choose from. You don't need the whole of Babeland's back section in your closet to enjoy kink.

A VERY GOOD PLACE TO START: IDEAS FOR FIRST-TIME KINKSTERS

Now, as a beginner, you don't have to call your local dungeon (how do you even find a dungeon? Is it on Google?). You can have plenty of kinky sex right at home. As I've hopefully plastered into your brain by now, kink is best served up slowly. Below are some fun places to start.

Role Play

Role play is the go-to when you're going to get kinky. It is easy to do and always a good time. Plus, I'd say like 98 percent of us have had a sexual fantasy where we were not us and our partners were not our partners. Role play gives you a chance to step outside of who you are every day and live out a fantasy.

Try a dom-sub role play as an aperitif to bondage. Grab a collar (or even a belt), and it puts the sub right into a submissive state. When you've got a collar on, you are someone's possession. It can really be as simple as that.

Spanking

You can add in some spanking, or try spanking in an entirely different scene. Spanking sends shock waves right through your whole body. It can add some *oomph* to otherwise standard sex.

Try having the spankee lean over a stack of pillows on the bed. Start soft and move up to more aggressive slaps. Let the person being spanked be in control of how hard you're hitting them. If he or she wants more, up the ante. If he or she wants you to hit softer or to stop, follow suit.

Anal Play

Buy an anal starter kit and begin with very small butt plugs before going to more advanced sizes. Always use lots of lube. Warm up the anus with a finger before inserting anything up there. You want the muscles to be relaxed. Getting ready for butt stuff can take days, weeks, or even months. Be careful with butts.

Don't be shy to try anal play with both you and your partner. One or both of you may enjoy it a lot. Sandra definitely suggests anal play if pegging is too intense.

But, if it isn't too intense, you can do pegging.

Pegging

Pegging is when you or your partner wears a strap-on with a dildo attached to it and gets in with the other person's bootylicious booty. In lieu of buying a ten-inch dildo, opt for the sweet spot of five to six inches. This, of course, comes after the anal training mentioned above. *Slow it down.*

Pegging gives you the opportunity to experience what it's like to have a dick. Gay, straight, bi, pan, or otherwise, this can be a huge turn-on for many women. Your partner will receive prostate stimulation (if he has a prostate), but that doesn't mean he or she needs a prostate to enjoy being fucked with a dildo.

The anus is full of nerves right at the opening. Some women/ people with vaginas can even have A-spot orgasms, where the internal clitoris is stimulated through the anus.*

Bondage

Tying each other up is a sexy-as-fuck way to explore different levels of control. You may be into having your feet, but not your hands, tied up. I personally only enjoy having my hands tied because if my feet are restrained, I get claustrophobic. Remember my panic attack?

Don't just grab string or a rope and go for it. Unless you're a trained knot tier or a Boy Scout,† opt for loose knots with a silk tie

---

* Another way you know kink is, like, so confusing. I have no idea which order to put these kink scenarios into. Some people would agree with my order, and others would not.

† Let's be real—no Girl Scout ever learns to tie knots, because the Scouts are some sexist bullshit.

(they come undone or can be cut if need be) or Velcro handcuffs. When you're trying bondage for the first time, the last thing you want is for someone to get stuck or lose circulation in their hands or feet.

Sensory Play

Sex is not just about getting your clit licked and touched. Engaging all of your senses—smell, touch, taste, sound, and sight—will take things to the next level. For real. Sensory play is a part of some BDSM play, but not all sensory play is BDSM. It can be sensual and romantic as well as dirty and nasty. It depends on how you engage in the play and what kinds of sensory experience you're looking for.

Hot Wax

Hot wax can be both erotic in pain play and part of a more sensual experience. For truly experienced BDSM practitioners, real hot wax that burns the fuck out of your skin might be what you want.

For beginners, do not do this. Do not just grab a candle from the storage closet and go ham. You will wind up in the ER. Claire Cavanah, cofounder of Babeland, gave me the lowdown on hot wax for *Glamour*. Use a massage candle, one that is specifically intended to be used for this purpose. It heats the wax to the right temperature so you can't burn your fucking skin off. Different candles burn to different temperatures, but most massage candles burn to a body-safe degree. It adds a layer of that kinky sadism, without exploring the pain aspect too much. Pouring something over your partner's skin is sexy; burning them maybe isn't. It's about the experience you want to have.

Sharp Play

No, I do not condone getting a box cutter from your old-school supplies kit and cutting your partner with it (though blood play is something some people are into). Get a blunted knife, a credit card, or a nail file. Place a T-shirt over your partner's eyes and run it across their skin. Sandra says the uncertainty in sensory play excites us.

If you want, you can grab a bunch of items and try out some different things on the skin and see what feels good. Danger without being too dangerous. It's all kinky and naughty. Sensations are sexy.

Kink is accessible for everyone. It doesn't make you a "bad girl" or "the girl you sleep with, not marry." You know, those old sayings I for one heard on every television show and in every novel I read growing up. If you're with someone who makes you feel like shit about yourself for wanting to step outside the vanilla sexually, don't hang out with that person anymore.

A person worth spending time with (and one worth fucking) is one who listens to your fantasies and respects them. He or she may not always want to try everything you're into, but he or she should appreciate your honesty and confidence. If you can't have a real-ass conversation, why are you even with that person? Ain't nobody got time for that.

Kink is a safe space to explore your boundaries and figure out new things you like. Use it as a learning experience and get on with your bad self.

Now, even with all the kinky and incredible sex in the world, you may still want to find love at some point. And sex and love are not mutually exclusive things. Who knew?

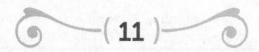

(11)

What's Love Got to Do
with Fucking?

Most people are terrible, but you absolutely do not have to
fuck them, love them, or date them.

Discerning your worth and coming to the conclusion that you
will no longer indulge total shitheads is a beautiful moment for any
woman. Once you decide you in no way would ever settle or compromise for something beneath you—and that in order for you to
consider a relationship of any kind, the person would have to be
simply extraordinary—you are liberated.

Even if you're not looking to settle down right now, understanding and respecting yourself in any romantic or sexual context
is a baller move. Putting an end to assholes infiltrating every area
of your life, and hole in your body, is a fascinating time in a person's
life. This is the phase in life when you are finally able to find something worth your time. If your patience for nonsense is nonexistent, the fuckwads weed themselves out very quickly.

You may have some issues with trust. You have likely been
fucked over a few times, but don't let someone amazing pass you
by just because you're trying not to get fucked over. This is where

you have to see the bigger picture—don't entertain douchebags, but don't assume every single person is a douchebag.

If you know how to discern a complete shit-for-brains dingus from a normal human, you know the only person getting into that heart of yours is going to be someone sensational. You, my dear, deserve nothing less than that. There are benefits to this whole love thing. The sex is a mix of hot and emotional all at once.

Love sex is the bomb, and it's something you need to have at some point in your life. I know this isn't a term I made up, but when I first experienced it, categorized it, and labeled it, I really thought I had. The fact of the matter is, love sex is something we women need to experience. It doesn't matter what your relationship status is—whether you're single, taken, poly, in an open relationship, looking for something casual, or whatever—love sex is an important part of becoming emotionally and sexually well rounded. It's about opening yourself up to vulnerability. That is where true strength is found—when you can open yourself up and let someone in without fear.

All the sex I had before my ex-boyfriend, and now my husband, was entirely selfish for me. The sex I had after my ex had been selfish sometimes, sometimes intimate, sometimes creative, and sometimes a mix of everything. Now, the sex I have with my husband is something even deeper, something I couldn't have had if I didn't allow myself that depth of intimacy.

Before actually being in love (real love) and giving an F about something, I wasn't beholden to anyone. I've always found power in sex, but the sex I'd had in the past was exclusively about empowerment through my own desire—the sex of a truly slutty girl who gives no fucks about pleasing anyone else. I used sexuality to conquer my own pleasure. This was amazing. It taught me what I liked. It showed me how to channel desire in a way that didn't include feelings. It was the potion for sexual empowerment that I craved and needed, like so many women who lack the tools to separate shame and sex, sex and emotion, emotion and pleasure.

After opening up my cold, black heart to another person, I understood sex in a whole new way. Love sex intertwines the power of pleasure and deep emotional connection, something I never thought was possible. Or maybe I knew it was possible, hypothetically, but was afraid of it. Nothing is scarier than letting your guard down when you're teetering on the edge of sexual empowerment and the hope of finding love. It's important to mention that I still felt that way, even when the relationship ended. I valued, and continue to value, the lessons I learned, regardless. You know. Maturity and shit. Just because you stop being in love with someone doesn't mean the lessons you learn about love, love sex, and passion go out the window. I don't know if I would have been able to allow my husband into my heart the way I had without the lessons of past love.

Before love sex, I found that sex was entirely a form of self-exploration. It was about the connection I had with myself. It didn't have the kind of emotional meaning that people talk about.

Of course, as the story goes with some great loves: *girl meets boy, boy sees girl every six months, boy grows beard, girl falls for boy's personality, boy and girl live happily ever after for three blissful years until the connection fades out and dies.*

Depressing as the ending sounds, don't lose sight of these very important lessons. And don't forget, I did find love again. True, lasting love. I'm married as fuck. It's kind of amazing how life can shape you if you let it.

Before I fell for my ex (and after), we fucked. A lot. I mean fucked. Not made love, fucked. We've had sex in every position, with every toy on the consumer market, in every location possible. It wasn't until a year or so into the relationship that we had love sex for the first time.

When I heard the term *lovemaking* or *making love,* I thought it was just another way of describing the sex I was having. I didn't realize there was a difference. My mom called sex *making love.* And I just thought she liked double-ended dildos and BDSM as much as I did. A rose by any other name, if you will.

But it was with this first great love that I figured out what it meant. I learned making love, or loving the person you're having sex with, is a different thing from fucking total strangers or a solid friend with benefits. It's not better or worse, it's just different.

In the past, I'd fucked a lot of guys (and a few choice ladies), but I'd never made love to any of them because that sounded legitimately terrible and scary.

I knew slow, passionate sex was real in a Hollywood sense, but I assumed it was something you really only saw in movies. I figured it would be very hard to vigorously flick my bean while keeping up this illusion of sweet tenderness. It did *not* make sense. Who would want to prolong orgasm instead of just making it happen?

I remember this one time when I was watching an '80s movie with my mom. I think Glenn Close (maybe Charlize Theron?) was in it. There was this scene where she and her love interest made love, or what I interpreted as making love (à la the silver screen). It was very slow, it was solely in missionary. After about 6.9 seconds, Glen/Charlize was crying out in orgasm. And then after it ended, she cried and her BF (or whatever) was lying there feeling very satisfied with himself.

I remember, even at the age of eleven, that this was stupid as fuck. All that slow, weird tenderness could never have provided an orgasm to the female body. You can't just stick a penis in a vagina and get there. There would have to be a lot more rubbing in that scenario. And then, how the fuck can it be slow if there is all that rubbing?

And why would I want that?

I wasn't really in love with any of the guys I slept with or dated. At various times, of course, I believed I was in love, but now that I know what love actually feels like and what it means, I understand that what I felt was infatuation at best and a cure for impending loneliness at worst. It was a crutch for a solitary existence, a way to fill a void.

Before my ex, I thought love was my fascination with different people and what they brought to my life. I thought it was just being adored. I loved being a trophy, something people were intrigued by and addicted to. It was some psycho shit.

It wasn't until I found someone who was both obsessed with me and challenged me that I realized what it meant to be in a healthy relationship. I found a person I really fucked with, someone who would stand up to me, called me on my bullshit, and still talked about our hypothetical children because he was so excited to have a future with me. And I never even puked once!

If any of my previous boyfriends had tried to make slow, passionate love to me, I would have likely had a full-blown panic attack and ended up on a stretcher. There is no way I would have allowed it or felt comfortable doing that.

I never felt safe enough with any of my past partners to let them have that kind of control during sex, to introduce such intense emotions into an act I thought I had complete power over. Everything was different in this relationship because of the introduction of real trust. I was willing to take the leap because I felt safe. I mean, come on. We're not even together anymore, and I can still appreciate this relationship and subsequent moment of sexual awakening for what it was: a growing experience of epic proportions. Even if someone fucks you over later, you can remember the good times if the relationship was a good one. Even good relationships end. My now husband can appreciate everything I learned from my last relationship and so can I. Sure, I was a bit jaded for a while, but I'm a stronger, more kickass woman than I've ever been before. For that, I have to truly thank my ex. I wouldn't be married to the man of my dreams if I'd never learned about love sex.

I liked (and still like) the animalistic nature of sex. I've always thought that the base grunting and selfish pleasure of sexuality was centering. What I didn't know, but happily learned, was that this element can exist in love sex, too. You never have to give up anything, ever. What a fucking concept!

So, the love sex. Yeah, yeah, I'm getting to that. It was the fall of 2016. We were about to have sex in my (truly disgusting and way too expensive) Brooklyn apartment.

"Let's fuck," I said, and I put my hand down his pants, amped up and ready to go.

We climbed into bed atop my purple sheets and took each other's clothes off between kisses. Kissing someone you're really into is like a fore-foreplay. I could feel his kisses from my lips all the way down to my vulva.

Everything is weird and magical when you really love someone. I wanted to lick the sweat from his armpits. It was intense attraction.

We left the lights on. I prefer to keep the lights on during sex. It makes me more present.

He laid me down on the bed and climbed on top of me. He touched my clit until I was wet. It was a different touch from what I was used to. It was slower, more measured. Though it made me nervous, I went with it, not about to turn down the chance to get laid.

It was when we started having penetrative sex that I became really confused. He moved slowly. He slid in and out at an alarmingly erotic pace. I could feel every inch of him. It made me insane. It made me uncomfortable. I grabbed that tight butt of his, trying to get him to pick up the pace.

"Calm down," he said.

I was out of my comfort zone. I was tensing up.

He just kissed me. I was desperate for some carnal, rabbit-level fucking, the sex I was used to—and comfortable—having.

Despite my instinct to get up and run, I gave in. I let it happen the way he wanted, slow and steady. I took a few deep breaths and closed my eyes, focusing on every sensation my body was feeling.

As I became enveloped in this intimate moment, my senses were suddenly heightened. I could feel every single nerve ending in my body light up. It was tantric. I was calm while the pleasure built inside me. I didn't fight it.

A combination of the nipple stimulation and slow thrusting led to something completely unexpected: my first intercourse-induced, G-spot orgasm.

We didn't even move from missionary position for the entire duration. (Side note: This wouldn't necessarily work for everyone).

My legs shook. My inner thighs were sore from clenching. My entire body was quivering. I hate to use the word *quivering* because it makes me want to hurl, but it's true. I was a quivering mess.

It was as close to being high on ecstasy as I could have been without popping some Molly/MDMA.

Now, I've had a shitload of sex with lots of different meat sacks, but this was different on so many levels. It was a complete departure from the very fabric of sex as I understood it.

This was the literal act of making love. It was the most intimate, vulnerable sex act I've ever experienced in my life. My heart was involved in a way that I didn't know was humanly possible. He fucked my heart, metaphorically. All the animalistic desire and white-hot internal fire I was accustomed to was still there, but muted like on a slow release. It was passionate and beautiful in a tender way that moved me to tears.

Yeah, I fucking cried. I cried. I did.

It's my job to be an authority on good ass, and I was over here crying because my boyfriend made love to me. Trust me, even after a breakup, you appreciate and miss that shit until you find it again. Sidenote: Totally did. And it gets even better.

I always thought sex was about getting fucked or fucking someone. It is a power exchange through partners, seeking orgasm. It was a basic, animalistic act we all crave and enjoy.

I was wrong.

When I told my girlfriends and sisters—all of whom are or have been in serious, loving relationships—about what happened, they laughed at me.

"Obviously, that's the best kind of sex," my little sister texted, adding on a bunch of upside-down smiley emojis because she's rude.

I expected everyone to be as flabbergasted as I was by this discovery. It felt like I'd unearthed some holy treasure and I needed to share it with the world.

To my dismay and embarrassment, apparently, I was the only person in a loving relationship who hadn't had passionate love sex.

Joke is on me, ladies. I get it. You can have this one.

THE IMPORTANCE OF LOVE SEX IN SEXUAL EXPLORATION

Love sex is the fucking bomb. Everyone needs to have it. Even us slutty, nasty women.

The point I'm trying to make is that this is not a kind of sex that should be feared, loathed, or actively prevented.

I want to be very clear here. I'm certainly not saying that love sex trumps all other sex. Hell, I've had sex that wasn't love sex (a.k.a. getting fucked really goddamn hard) since this sexy experience, and it's been unbelievable. Your sex threshold is wide. It is vast. You can have all of that kinky BDSM sex we talked about and have love sex. Your BDSM sex might be love sex, who knows?

As long as you're having it safely, I totally encourage you to get as much penis/vagina as your heart desires in whatever form and orifices you choose. Just use a condom and don't use sex as a way to boost your self-esteem or to fill a tragic void of self-loathing.

We need to use sex as a way to learn about ourselves and what brings us pleasure. It is in your control. Love sex isn't a weaker form of sex just because it has an underlying element of tenderness. Sex, in all its forms, is fantastic. There is no right or wrong way to do it. It's all about what makes you feel good.

For me, love sex was terrain unmastered or even imagined. It turned into an exploration into the possibilities of sex. It was a great foray into a world that had been unknown to me.

In my personal experience, I've found that empowered slutty women fear passion and feelings. We've all been there, trying to avoid any emotional connection when it comes to fucking in order to stave off any actual bonding. Technically, your brain can't even tell the difference between a partner and casual sex. An orgasm releases oxytocin (the love hormone) and creates a false sense of closeness.

If you stave off bonding, the sex remains casual, and you are ultimately in control of the situation. Society has programmed us to equate desire with emotion, and biology has smothered us with love hormones to confuse us even further.

These experiences are not black and white. Sex can be emotional, emotionless, semi-emotional, and so on. Love sex is about opening yourself up to emotional sex in the right setting, with the right person. It starts with trust. Once you have trust, you can form love. Once you have love, you can be vulnerable without fear.

Love sex is about allowing yourself to traverse the boundaries of passion with the *right* person. Even if that person isn't the right person forever. Sometimes the right person is the right person now, in the moment, in this time in your life. If you choose a good person and open your heart to love, the possibilities are endless. Being with the right person doesn't hinder your sexuality. It doesn't make you less of a slutty girl. I promise. It doesn't make sex less dirty or kinky or fun.

It just creates a safe space, and that safe space makes sexual vulnerability possible. You don't need to be sexually vulnerable every time you fuck someone, but it helps to know it's possible.

PORN AND ITS INFLUENCE
ON THE SEX WE HAVE

All our views on sex are shaped by the media we consume, and none is so transcendent as pornography. It all comes back to porn every single time, doesn't it? I thought I knew everything about sex at twenty years old. I was like, "I like to get fucked! Hard!" It's not so surprising. I watched a lot of hard-core porn. I didn't have context. I thought I wanted to experience sex like a porn star: as a submissive, getting railed until sunrise. It looked awesome on film, and it felt good in practice. So this was a safe space for me. It worked.

When it comes to kids and education, porn is precarious because of the way it affects sexual understanding in society. When we're exposed to heavy, hard-core sexual imagery as kids, we don't wind up free of its influence. Not everyone is totally self-aware and unaffected by what they see in any projected form of media, especially pornos. Myself included.

As it turns out, I also really like slow, intimate sex. I didn't fully comprehend the effect my porn consumption had on my sexual desire until I had sex that departed from those erotic constructs. It's not inherently porn's fault. Porn is entertainment. Porn isn't meant to be the foundational education of a young person's sexual education. But as they say, tough shit. Porn is how we learn about sex. No one else wants to teach us. *Gang Bang Schoolgirl Nurses XIII* is our *Odyssey*.

Experiencing different types of sex as an adult is how we move away from the ideas of sex we've been fed through porn. It wasn't until I had love sex that I truly understood that smutty, dirty sex was not the *only* way sex can be enjoyed. It isn't that I don't enjoy porn-style sex sometimes, it's that it was the only sex I thought existed. When you see nothing other than threesomes and fisting scenes, why would you intuitively know other sex exists?

Do not get me wrong on the whole porn thing. I love porn. I really do. It's true that most of the mainstream stuff is problematic in some form or another. The industry is sexist, many scenes blatantly exploit the "sexy" idea of coercing women into sex when they don't want to, because ultimately the mainstream shit is created for men. Once we have more female porn makers, we'll see a true revolution in female pleasure and the understanding of what women want in bed. I still watch and enjoy it. There is nothing wrong with watching porn. As long as you recognize the issues and understand that it is a fantasy and you or your partner are not allowing porn to overtake your sex life, you should watch or not watch as much porn as you want. You're an adult person. Do what you want.

Obviously, issues do arise. There are instances where porn can force you or your partner out of the bedroom. I had a friend who told me that she and her girlfriend rarely had sex anymore because she was so overstimulated by porn. She could only have an orgasm if one of her videos was on. Their real sex life took a back seat.

While these "bad" instances are not super common, we have to stop forcing ourselves on either side of the pro-porn/anti-porn gate and recognize it has its merits and deficiencies. While fun and highly stimulating, porn can present problems that negatively affect both you and those around you. This should be actively fought against and checked in a hot second if it starts happening to you.

If you take precautions and use porn in a healthy manner, you really have nothing to fear. Just be aware of your pornographic consumption. Keep tabs on it. As long as you are approaching it in a logical manner and considering your partner's needs and feelings, it's normal.

How does this relate to love sex, Gigi? You're so obsessed with porn.

We see sex portrayed in these sexy and dirty ways, and that's actually all we really know. Our personal fantasies and what we consider erotic become imbued with these images we see en masse.

We have to marry reality with the RedTube fantasies that have saturated our ideas of sex. I enjoy porn but have to recognize the negative effects it can have if it's not consumed responsibly. Make sense?

The only way we get around the porn fiasco is by educating people. We have to teach people about sex and what it means to have good, consensual sex. We don't need to get rid of porn; porn just can't be the only thing we ever see.

Not all sex has to be raunchy. Not all sex has to end with a gang bang and a come shot. These are things we'd understand if we were taught about pleasure, about the emotionality that can come of sex, about the trust that can be fostered between two partners. We're fucked up about sex because we don't know any better. We think if it's not some super-loud, multi-orgasmic, screaming squirt fest, it isn't up to par.

Sex can be experienced and enjoyed in a variety of ways that are both erotic, healthy, and even passionate. This means making a conscious departure from what we see on Pornhub's most-viewed list and actually try to experience sex in its many shapes and forms, including love sex.

LOVE SEX: THE CONNECTION OF MIND AND BODY

We have to remember that there is no wrong way to have sex. Or I guess we have to learn that in the first place. There is no wrong way to experience sexuality. Sex comes in all shapes and forms. It can be hot, dirty, and dangerously sexy, but it can also be slow, sweet, and passionate. It can be every single adjective all at the same time or have no descriptors at all. It can be penetrative, oral, masturbating together, or solo. You have to experience (or at least appreciate) sex in all its forms to fully understand its magnitude. The love sex I have with my husband is pretty goddamn raunchy, but it's still love sex. The intention is there. The kissing and snuggles post calling me a dirty whore are part of the whole experience. I dig it.

Love sex may not be the most raunchy sex you ever have, but it will teach you some shit about yourself. It teaches you about your capacity for expansive feeling and thinking. Since so many of us have learned about sex through the lens of porn and movies, having love sex can open our eyes to a whole new way of thinking—it is natural, but it feels unusual because of our lack of exposure.

Love sex forces you to focus on the act itself and its ability to have meaning in certain contexts. In many other sexual situations, you have the ability to zone out. You don't have to think about this other person as you are exerting all your effort on the act of fucking.

When you have love sex, there is no escaping your thoughts, your mind, and your body. You have to look at every inch of yourself, you have to feel every inch of yourself. It makes you stronger while, at the same time, making you vulnerable.

Allowing yourself to be vulnerable takes strength. You're opening yourself up to another person, exposing your soul. It is raw and open. You are not weak. Your trust for the person you're with has simply surpassed all the walls you've built around yourself.

We spend so much time protecting our hearts, but it takes a real strength of character to let yourself be susceptible to pain or loss—and to learn from the loss of that person if it happens one day.

You can have as much sex as you want in any way that you want, but be open to all of it—if only intellectually. Otherwise, how can you know what you really want? I spent the whole of my sexual maturation thinking sex was my liberation, and yet I had no idea the depths of which it could be experienced.

Sex is physical, but it has the capability to be so much more than that. Sex can be physical, emotional, and spiritual. It is an opportunity to be completely connected with your partner. Being able to have that with someone is a great thing, even if the relationship itself doesn't last forever. (We'll get more into the intricacies of heartbreak later.)

Love and the sex you have while in love opens your mind to a whole new way of seeing yourself, the world, and the possibilities of pleasure.

Love sex is not denied to us nasty women. You don't damage your chance of finding love by knowing what you deserve and accepting nothing less. Quite the opposite, in fact. Our sexual exploration and freedom is what leads us to experience love sex on a much more profound level than others might. Through learning what you want and empowering yourself through your sexuality, you have opened the door to the full range of possibilities in both sex and love.

When you're a proud, empowered female, it is easy to fear giving up your sexual freedom, but there is nothing stunting about the experience of falling in love if love is what you want. Embracing your true power as a woman means letting go of what society expects of you and not giving a fuck what people think of your happiness.

It's about taking away the negative connotations of what it means to be a woman who likes sex and has it however she wants. You're not having sex with multiple people because you have low self-esteem or don't have standards. You're not choosing not to have sex because you're a prude. You're having sex the way you want because you answer to no one but yourself.

Being sexually liberated in a way that feels right to you is how you find your strength.

You can kick ass at life only when you truly know and accept yourself. It can only happen when you accept the love you deserve— even if that love is the love you have for yourself entirely.

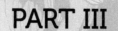

PART III

Let Me Save You the Trouble:
Finding the Love You Deserve

Once a Cheater

Before we get into the ~~nuts and bolts~~ dildos and clit vibes of finding love, we have to chat about some of the shit we go through before we're ready for that kind of love. Finding a fabulous relationship means experiencing a lot of difficult situations and having them explode right in your face, much like an unexpected jizz-gasm from a guy you just started seeing and don't even like that much.

Nothing epitomizes the emotional volcanic diarrhea explosion of horrid relationships like cheating. So let's talk a little bit about cheating. Let's start with me—a cheated-on cheater. What a world.

I was the other woman when I was nineteen. Following that, I cheated on every partner I'd ever had. Cheating exists wherever there is self-loathing, dissatisfaction in the relationships (sexually and/or emotionally), and insecurity. Many a young woman finds self-loathing to be a regular companion on her personal life journey, and I had a lot of that. I cheated because I didn't know what else to do. I was terrified of being the one who got hurt after being burned that first time, so I did the hurting.

Let me take you on a little trip down memory lane. The beginning of it all. To the time in my life when I fell in love with a pathological cheater—the experience with cheating that set me on the path to being a cheater myself. I promise all that self-loathing stuff will make sense. I know about this shit because I lived it.

Tessa, my skinny, every-finger-ring-toting college roommate, introduced me to Isaac when I was a freshman in college. She was almost manic in her excitement about this love match, and she generally doesn't get excited about anything (she's from LA; it's not her fault). She enthusiastically informed me that we were so similar: gregarious, emotive, slightly insane.

Isaac was dark-haired with an earring and miscellaneous tattoos. He had two roosters inked into his sides and also a lamppost haphazardly placed in there somewhere—two cocks and a lamppost. He wasn't traditionally attractive. What he really had was charisma. When he spoke, people were drawn to him. He had a way of making you feel important, like you were the only person in the world.

Instantly, a chemical, animalistic attraction kicked in for us both. From the moment he said hello, he didn't take his eyes off me. His laugh gave me goose bumps and made my clit buzz.

Isaac's charms were like an infectious disease; one person in the room caught the bug and then passed it on to someone else. Pretty soon everyone was lapping up what he was serving, myself included.

I don't know how much we actually spoke that evening, but I sensed that our bodies needed to be touching. Naked.

As our group left the pregame to go out for the night, Isaac and I redirected the cab we were sharing to go home and strip each other's clothes off in my extra-long twin bed. I had my first orgasm with another person that night. That oxytocin, it's like a drug. I became an addict; I needed my next hit.

We were quite a pair. Two hedonists with a penchant for Jim

Beam and bad decisions. The morning after we first had (mind-blowing) sex and went about our days, we simultaneously made our Facebook statuses, "[Insert name] is a hot mess." It was Wi-Fi-enabled cosmic fate.

We got close quickly, spending our days in bed hungover and our nights drinking cheap whiskey and having lots of sex. Not only was he the first person to get me off during P-in-the-V sex, he was also the first person to ever go down on me. It was like crack.

At bars and clubs, we spent entire nights wrapped around each other. I felt like I had won the big prize. On Isaac's arm, I absorbed his energy. I became the most interesting person in the room, too.

Our foundation was sex, but Isaac soon grew to be more than someone I was just fucking. He became the center of my world. We talked about everything. Well, with one exception—his girlfriend back home.

There is no worse agony than being the side chick. You are the half-loved one. You're the one who is not good enough. You're never "the One." You're never the priority. Eventually, you forget what it's like to be treated as a human being who's even deserving of love. The list of what is important to you gets sidetracked by bullshit.

I wasn't some innocent victim. I knew Isaac had a serious girlfriend before I slept with him, but I don't think that either one of us even considered that a reason to avoid hooking up. We were nineteen, an age where you lack big-picture thinking and are almost always drunk (refer to chapter 3 on all the stupid drunk shit we do when we don't know who we are). I knew I was supposed to care, but I didn't care enough.

The weight of the affair didn't set in until I fell in love with him—which I did quickly and violently. *Great job, Gigi. I'm sure this story is going to end up happily,* said no one ever.

The inevitable happened, of course: I became every cliché side chick. Thinking I was different and special . . . knowing in my bones that we would end up together. But I wasn't different. I wound up so absorbed in his charms that he was even able to convince me to edit most of his college papers (add *tutor* to the growing list of talents I was offering up with no remuneration). I pretended his girlfriend didn't exist and refused to speak of her, forbidding Tessa and our other friends from broaching the subject, too. I was in a constant state of frenzy, wrapped up in the game of winning him, while battling an overwhelming sense of impermanence.

It was a concoction of self-preservation and self-loathing: the deadly makeup of the side chick's psyche.

For all my acting like a pathetic idiot, I wasn't clueless. I knew things weren't right. I was aware that this was a shitshow. Our bond was somehow growing both deeper and weaker at the same time. I became desperate for his affection and more insecure about our arrangement. *If I just show him how amazing and funny and gorgeous I am, he'll eventually wake up and realize that I'm the one for him, right?* Of course, that's never how it goes. He wanted to have his cake and eat it, too.

If you're a crappy-enough person to juggle two women in the first place (without consent), why would you suddenly break up with one of them when you could keep a girlfriend at school and another back home? It's simple logic.

Everything came to a head one morning in early April. Tessa informed me that Isaac's girlfriend was in town and that the whole crew was getting together for lunch.

Isaac hadn't told me about her visit, obviously. I was terrified by how horrible I felt. With my heart like a fragile balloon, I spent the entire day in bed, unable to move. I didn't even cry, instead just lying there in agony.

Isaac and I continued sleeping together sporadically for a few weeks after, but the whole thing felt poisoned. The bubble had burst. The harsh reality of the situation was beyond plausible deniability.

One night at a club, we did too much cocaine and screamed at each other, but there was no grand finale or fiery crescendo. The only thing that came out of that was an aggravated anxiety disorder that I'm still dealing with to this day.

The novelty of the whole had faded. It had become tired. Isaac wasn't willing to slow down and commit to me (not that I had the balls to ask him), and I'd grown worn out from waiting. Where spending time with him had once given me butterflies in my stomach, now it just made me sad.

The texts were fewer and further between, until they stopped coming altogether. I started sleeping with some other guy and then another; Isaac started sleeping with other women, too—and notably continued dating his girlfriend.

When I started writing about this event in articles all around the internet (including my blog in 2013—there really is no limit to how embarrassing I can be), I felt worse for myself than his girlfriend. I knew I should take full responsibility for my part in the affair, but the girlfriend was never real to me. She was just a cartoon character with a pixie cut. I feel differently about that now. Having done enough cheating myself, I have the ability to see everything from both sides.

Here is what I learned about side chicks: Being the side chick means you're painted as a vile harlot who is out to ruin the lives of committed, "good" women. Conveniently exempted from this stigma: the person who chose to cheat on this "good woman." Despite the reputation, the side chick is rarely malicious. She isn't sleeping with another woman's boyfriend or husband or girlfriend or wife or partner because she's a terrible, home-wrecking nutjob. She's in so deep that the consequences don't matter. She doesn't want to be a side chick. She wants to be the only chick. The only problem is that she, like many women, chose to love a jerk.

Looking back on what I had with Isaac, I can see how glaringly wrong it all was. It felt like love, but it wasn't. Love lifts you up. It makes you feel whole, happy, confident, and adored. It doesn't eat away at you like bacteria.

In the same vein, there is a strange sense of displacement when you are the person who does the cheating. It can be an out-of-body experience. A couple of years later, I was dating a DJ with DEAD-MAU5 tattooed to his arm and a Union Jack on the back of his neck.* He was a really nice guy in a lot of ways and a complete fuckwad in others—you know, like 99 percent of the human race.

I never felt secure in my relationship with him. I was constantly, desperately trying to make him love me. He would be wonderful to me, and then do things that undermined our relationship in such a low-key but fundamental way that I could never predict or understand where we stood. One amazing example of the mind-fuck that was this relationship comes to the forefront every time I talk about this Top-40s piece of shit.

He asked if I'd help him move into his new apartment. His mom and sister would be there. I had never met them. I was excited and nervous. It made me feel like a model girlfriend to show his

---

* I clearly had a thing for guys with stupid-as-fuck tattoos. My taste was impeccable!

mom and sister that I was willing to take off from work and help my boyfriend move into his apartment.

When I arrived, my boyfriend was off getting the moving van. I was alone with his mom and sister. After about five minutes of polite conversation, it dawned on me—they had never heard of me. Neither one of them knew who I was. They had never heard my name before. My boyfriend had let me take off work to come to his apartment to help him move. And he hadn't even told his family that I was his girlfriend. They didn't even know he had a girlfriend. We had been dating for seven months. I had one of my friends call me and pretend there was a family emergency and left before he came back with the moving van.

We got into a fight that ended with me apologizing for expecting him to share his personal life with his family, as if this were a reasonable thing. I told him I was sorry for what happened. He managed to make me feel like this was entirely my fault.

I cheated on him throughout our relationship, at different times with different random people. We would get into a fight. He'd make me feel like shit about myself. I'd cheat. He'd ditch me for his friends. I wouldn't say anything to him. I would get blackout drunk. I'd cheat.

One night, he told me he wanted to hang out with one of his friends. His friend who was also his ex-girlfriend. I wasn't invited. I didn't think I had a right to complain or to say no. So I punished him in my own way. I had a party at my friend's apartment in Rogers Park. I made out with a hot firefighter and cried into his mouth out of guilt and muted rage. Later that same night, completely shithoused, I had sex with one of my friends in the living room, and apparently my little sister was on the couch, witnessing the whole thing. She is basically forever traumatized, and we joke about what a garbage person I was to this very day. I am nothing if not classy.

I'm not saying that my cheating on my DJ boyfriend was entirely his fault, because my unhappiness, lack of self-worth, and the constant questions played a significant role in my choices. I was deeply unhappy, obsessed with him, and afraid of being alone. It was my fault for cheating; his fault was being a terrible boyfriend. He didn't make me do anything, but he certainly didn't make me happy or feel safe in any way.

This pattern of behavior continued into the rest of my relationships for many years to follow. My lack of personal accountability coupled with crippling self-loathing, burgeoning alcoholism, and terrible taste in romantic partners made me an epic cheater. I had masterfully crafted a pocketful of excuses for my behavior.

Wherever there is cheating, there is a lack of love for yourself. The two go hand in hand. They are like tequila and soda—a perfect match and deadly combination. Whether you are the perpetrator, the accomplice, or the one staying in a relationship with a cheater, there is bountiful and visceral despair. Let's take a quick moment to clarify that I'm talking about women in their twenties and thirties here. I don't have enough experience with therapy to make a blanket judgment call on married couples who have been together for years on end. I'll let experts like Esther Perel and Tammy Nelson take the reins on that one. But, for us dumb AF millennials and Gen Z-ers, it's a nightmare of personal self-hatred up in this bitch.

This despair likely pertains to men as well, but women are a special brand of cheaters. Blame society, blame the way we're wired by ideas of gender, blame whatever you like. It doesn't make it less true. If you cheat, you are compensating for a lack of self-love and self-worth in some way or another. You are sabotaging the relationship, and the reasons are probably so fucking complicated that you can't even draw them out. Cheating is the Ebola virus of love. It eats you up from the inside, is highly contagious, and kills pretty much anyone it comes in contact with.

WHY WE CHEAT AND WHAT IT MEANS

This is what I know.

You cannot cheat on someone you truly love. You cannot. You can't. It is not possible.

This doesn't mean you don't care about them. For a woman, it doesn't mean you don't want your partner to be happy. You may not know what else to do but cheat when the relationship is dysfunctional and you're flailing around, attempting to hold it together. You want the control when you have so little. You have so little happiness that you find it in small, insignificant moments of infidelity. You can love them, but you don't love them in a healthy way. It's not so much about loving them "enough" but loving them in the right way. You don't. If you love your partner the way they deserve to be loved, you won't cheat. If they love you the way you should be loved, they will not cheat on you. And it's more complicated still. If you have a happy, healthy relationship, an egalitarian relationship, you won't cheat. Why would you? Cheating is a symptom of imbalance and general discontent.

Love is as much about respect as it is about passion and romance. If you don't have enough respect for your partner not to cheat, you shouldn't be in that relationship. It goes both ways. Think about what it takes to cheat on someone. You have to flirt with the person you're about to cheat with, ask them to go somewhere private, take off each other's clothes, (hopefully) put a condom on (internal or external), and then put your penis in someone or put someone's penis in you (being heteronormative here, but this obviously applies to all kinds of couples) or touch someone in a sexual way.

This is not like, "Oops, my vulva just accidentally touched your mouth." Or, "Oh-Em-Gee, my penis just fell into her vagina! My bad!" or "IDK how I wound up fingering a woman who was not my wife, but hey."

The "I'm so sorry! It just happened!" excuse is not a fucking excuse. Don't try to tell me that this was a mistake. A mistake is dropping your phone and cracking the screen. A mistake is the barista using whole milk instead of 2 percent. A mistake is wearing bright blue underwear with a thin heather-gray dress. A mistake is overcooking the chicken. Fucking someone is not a mistake. Get the fuck out of here with that shit.

I am calling out every single person out there (myself included) who has handed out some nonsensical bullshit excuse for cheating, and every single asshole who has accepted one. I should know. I have cheated, I have been cheated on, and I've been a side chick. I've wanted power, and I've taken power. I've been powerless and fucked strangers instead of talking it out with my person. My ex got hand jobs from sex workers in seedy massage parlors when we fought.

There is some other stuff that a lot of people don't get when it comes to cheating, shit that is pretty apparent from the stories I shared. Cheating is a lot less about the person you cheat on and a lot more about you, the person who does the cheating. Cheating is not a malicious act for most women. I can't definitively say the same about men, but women I know. I'm sure for many guys, their cheating isn't intended to be hurtful, but from what I've seen from readers and clients alike, cheating is about control, which manifests in very different ways based on gender. It's an ego boost for many of us, but it isn't the same type of ego boost. It makes men feel good about themselves—like they have the power in the relationship. It can often show how women are disposable and easily manipulated. Now, that has malicious undertones, to be sure.

For many women, it's an ego boost that ends in profound guilt. It's not even about getting the ego boost but is more geared toward getting a small amount of love in any way we can. Sad? Yeah, it is. Not that it stops us, obviously. We're totally still cheaters and do it all the time.

It's incredible and depressing how gender norms warp the ways we think and feel about cheating, in general and in our own personal lives. Men have more power than women in this world, and being able to exercise that power and show a woman her supposed worth and place are a part of a larger understood social narrative that we live and die by. Please refer to part 1 of this book in case you missed it.

Yes, don't get all eye-roll-y on me. I am talking about the Patriarchy again. In a society where women are conditioned to feel guilt, to cater to feelings of others, and be emotional caretakers, it only makes sense that cheating would be less about causing hurt and more about grasping at the small moments of control we have over our lives—and then drowning in guilt. For most women, anyway. I rarely felt guilty when I cheated myself. I felt like I was sticking it to the system. I know there are women who have this same remorselessness about cheating. It's not like we're all wounded birds just looking for love. Come on. By being remorseless and an all-in-all giant douchebag, I took on that gendered "male" role. How about that for a fucked-up situation? Being the "man" in the power structure of any given relationship somehow made me the "better" one? Like?

As many before me (and after me), I cheated as a quiet act of resistance to being treated poorly in relationships. I saw it as my own secret "Fuck you." Even then, it was about me. I was the one so insecure in my relationship that I didn't know how to communicate my own unhappiness. I didn't care enough about myself to get out of the relationship. I didn't do anything to help fix the situation before I went outside of it.

As noted, people don't cheat in happy, secure relationships. Cheating is not the problem; cheating is a symptom of deeper, fatal relationship problems. People cheat when they are deeply insecure. People cheat when they feel trapped and suffocated, even when that entrapment was by their own design. People cheat when they don't trust their partner not to cheat first. You do the destroying so that the other person needn't bother. You sabotage the whole thing, walling off your heart from the wreckage so as to avoid getting hurt.

Cheating is a way to temporarily relieve some of the pain you have in a shitty relationship. For many of us ladies, it's those fleeting feelings of worthiness we chase after when there is no source for it at home. It's a quick fix to a much bigger problem. It's like drinking vodka to alleviate anxiety; you feel better in the moment, but much worse the next day once the shame sets in.

In my first few years after moving to New York City, I was dating an abusive man in his late thirties. I was twenty-one, and like most twenty-one-year-olds, I was a fucking moron. He would refer to himself as "Daddy" in the third person and would regularly put me down about my studies, my internships, my nannying jobs, and my cheap Zara-sale-rack clothes. He had a lot of money, and I had no money. I cheated on him because I needed to feel a sense of control over my life, one I couldn't have while with him. I figured if I cheated on him after drinking enough watered-down vodka at the club, he couldn't possibly be the bad guy in the relationship because I had made myself a bad guy, too. I deluded myself into thinking that the abuse wasn't abuse because I was a shitty partner, too. We both had our flaws, right?

Whether you are a man, woman, or neither, cheating is not about sex; it's about control. It isn't about pleasure, even if there are orgasms involved. The orgasms are momentary bliss in an otherwise thoroughly fucked-up situation. Like taking drugs, it feels good in the moment, and it has an epically shitty come-down.

Cheating is a dealbreaker.

Countless sex therapists and other totally respectable and brilliant authorities have told me that they've seen affairs save marriages. That it was something that "needed to happen to bring a couple back together." I've been told affairs have the power to kick a couple's ass into shape and start healing their relationship.

Hahahahahahahaha

Hahahahahahhahahahahahaha

Ahahahaha

Ahah

Ha.

No.

Fuck that. You can take that notion, write it on a piece of paper, and shove it up your ass. You know, respectfully. If cheating "had to happen" to make you fix your shitty relationship, you should evaluate your fucking priorities. How shitty does a relationship have to be that you need to betray your partner to open your fucking eyes? Fuck no.

If you cheat on someone, you have to end the relationship because there is really no coming back from it. Cheating is saying, "I don't love you. I don't respect you. Your happiness is not important."

Maybe you think you can forgive and move on; Lord knows plenty of experts have told me you can, but I think that you break something when you cheat that can't be fixed. The memory will always be there. It will always be there between you, and you will always know what the other person is capable of doing. You will be completely aware that this person has it in them to sleep with someone else. Forever.

Frankly, you deserve better than that shit. You need to believe that you deserve better than that shit. We need to stop trying to fix what is not worth fixing and instead equip ourselves with enough fucking self-respect to walk away from a toxic, bullshit relationship and move on. If a professional tells you that it's better to try to fix a relationship with someone who cheated than it is to build something healthy with a person who gives enough of a fuck not to do it, stop giving that person money. If you walk away from the relationship, you'd stop having a reason to go to therapy. There goes the therapist's paycheck. I'm not saying it's a conspiracy theory, but if the butt plug fits . . .

Why try to fix something *that* broken? A relationship you really deserve is not one built on a bed of distrust. You don't have to settle for someone who cheats on you.

ONCE A CHEATER IS NOT ALWAYS A CHEATER

For those of you who have cheated or are with someone who cheated in the past with other girlfriends or boyfriends or people, you should know that the old saying is a total lie. It's a lie in the same way that saying that cheating is forgivable is a lie. Take it from someone who seriously knows, you aren't always a cheater just because you have a past with it. I may shit all over cheating, but it doesn't mean the behavior is irredeemable. The relationship may be tanked, but you as a human being, are not.

Cheating can be a compulsion, sure. You shouldn't be in a relationship at all if you are pathologically cheating, and you shouldn't be with someone who makes it known that they've cheated in the past and can't promise it won't happen again in this new relationship.* If you believe you have compulsory cheating behavior, that is something you need to work on with yourself and your therapist. You have a problem that no amount of dating is going to fix. You have to fix yourself if you want to have a relationship that is healthy and secure. That is, after all, what it takes to not cheat. You have to love yourself and be willing to accept happiness and love from someone else. You need to work on your own shit so you don't keep fucking up your own life. But that is 100 percent something you are capable of doing.

If you're stable, grounded, and comfortable with yourself, you'll be able to function in a relationship without straying. You won't feel the need if the relationship is healthy and you love yourself. If you believe in your heart that you deserve a happy life, you won't fuck up your life. It's a lot simpler than we make it out to be. If the relationship becomes toxic, you need to have the self-worth to walk away.

You stop cheating when you find someone you fuck with enough

---

* That sure sounds like someone making up really stupid excuses for their very real intention to seek ass elsewhere!

to commit to and fuck with yourself enough to do right by the person you love. You stop cheating when you feel like you can say, "I'm unhappy with X. Can we work on this?" without fear of being admonished by your supposed boo. You have to date someone you actually care about and respect as a person, someone who fulfills you and positively impacts your life. Someone you fucking trust. Someone who satisfies you sexually or, if not, is willing to try sexual variety and new things. Someone who would be willing to explore sexual non-monogamy or another form of relationship if it means making you both happier overall.

The self-love stuff has to happen before all the other happiness can evolve and grow. Don't go out and try to find someone to fix you. No one is going to fix you but you. I know the popular mind-set is: *Accept me for who I am or fuck off!* And while I fully subscribe to you being true to yourself and being the magical queen that you are, pulling some fuckgirl shit is not cute. If who you are is a shitty fucking person, you need to check yourself. We'll get more into that in following chapters. I'm here to help you have better sex and a better life. I don't give a fuck about coddling your feelings, and neither should you. We're here to grow, so let's grow.

WHEN CHEATING *ISN'T* A DEALBREAKER

When I hit Isaac up on Facebook Messenger to get his permission to use his real name for this book, he told me that he's no longer cheating on everyone with a vengeance, but rather is up front about his actions and preferences in any relationship or dating situation.

"I'm no longer a cheater. I tell everyone that I sleep with that I have six girlfriends before I sleep with them."

"Hey, ethical non-monogamy is perfectly acceptable as long as you're not lying," I told him. That is so goddamn rad!

As we've covered at length, a relationship should be about trust and respect. If those things exist in your relationship, whatever the specified dynamic, that is fabulous. Trust is critical. If you are lying to your partner about sleeping with and/or dating other people, that is cheating. It is lying. Betrayal is not the new black, baby. If your relationship with someone is consensually open, polyamorous, and the like, it's not cheating. If you've discussed these parameters and everyone in the relationship is comfortable and excited about them, you're good. Every single relationship is different. Monogamy doesn't work for everyone; it is just the most common type of relationship. It's just another lie. Monogamy is a kind of relationship you can choose; that doesn't mean it needs to be the default relationship we all aspire to be in. That sounds like some brainwashed Beaver Cleaver bullshit to me.

There is nothing wrong with being in an open relationship if that's what you want. If you want that, don't let another person on this, the planet Earth, tell you there is anything wrong with that. We are so over the judgmental, pandering, monogamy-only shitstorm as fully developed nasty women. We are ready for a new phase, thank you. I sat down with fellow sex writer Sophie Saint Thomas to talk about her fabulously well-managed and glam AF, non-monogamous lifestyle. She told me that being non-monogamous was difficult for her last partner. He wanted traditional monogamy. This wasn't something she could offer, as being non-monogamous is just a part of who she is as a person. She was up front about what she needed in the relationship and gave him an opportunity to be with her under these conditions. There was no lying involved. As long as you're honest about who you are and what you want out of a relationship, and you go about it in an ethical way, there is nothing wrong with breaking the traditional mold and finding a setup that fits your needs. Traditional is not synonymous with *good* or *better*. Are some people going to be dicks about your not wanting one partner forever until you die and are dead? Probably. People don't know how to deal with things that don't look the way they're used to—the way the mainstream media and whitewashed ideals have plopped them out. Fuck those people. They can either catch up or eat your dust as you ride off on your magical unicorn with your two sexy lovers.

However, be wary of an arrangement that is only to please your partner. This is something to consider if you're new to an open or poly lifestyle (or are considering it). A big problem can arise in open or poly relationships when one partner wants to be open and the other partner agrees in order to stay in the relationship. That isn't healthy. That is missing the point entirely. If you're "allowing" someone to sleep with other people because they won't be with you under the circumstances that make you comfortable, don't be in that relationship. Everyone in a relationship has the right to feel happy and fulfilled. To piggyback on that, poly or open does not mean cheating isn't possible. If you sleep with someone (or fool around with, whatever) without your partner's consent, lie to your partner about who you are dating or sleeping with, etc., etc., guess what? THAT IS STILL CHEATING! Esther Perel says in her book *The State of Affairs* that cheating not only happens in open relationships, it's quite common. So, don't think you're getting off free just because you're open. There are still boundaries and respect that need to be taken into account.

If an open relationship is what you want, that is fucking awesome. I'm so here for it. We should all be here for it. Relationships look and function differently for different people. It's time we stop pretending one "style" fits us all. That's like saying my lime-green, seven-inch strap-on is going to be the fantasy of the whole human race. That is just not at all true. Who the fuck has a right to judge you and what makes you happy? As long as all parties involved are comfortable and happy with the relationship arrangement, you have to do you. Fuck everyone else and their "Wow. But how can you really love someone if you have sex with other people?" pig-headed nonsense. They can shove it up their own ass—and not in the good, anal-beads kind of way.

I briefly had a podcast about sex and relationships with my ex (which, in retrospect was not one of my better ideas, actually). We interviewed my married friends Han and Matt. They are in a great, stable, polyamorous marriage, full of communication and trust. They are goals, really. They each have relationships outside of the marriage. When I last saw them, Matt had recently gone to Florida to visit his girlfriend of two years and came back with painted toenails. Just recently, Han broke up with their long-term boyfriend and girlfriend. The couple they were dating were married to each other. The evidence of all of these romantic endeavors is readily available on their social media profiles. They hide nothing because there is nothing to hide.

Han and Matt both actively date on a variety of apps and websites, where they are up front with potential new partners about their poly status. They coordinate their schedules so that one of them is out with friends if the other wants to bring a date home. This is what makes them happy. When I asked them how they manage to keep up with so many liaisons while maintaining a marriage and their careers, Matt looked at me, rather puzzled. "I've always prioritized relationships over everything," he said.

They put each other first and value each other. Some poly couples don't believe in hierarchies, wherein there is a primary partner, and others do. No one setup is superior to the other. Han and Matt are married and have relationships with other people. They told me that there are certainly issues with jealousy and, as with any relationship, problems arise. They are able to overcome any hurdle because they respect and love each other enough to be open and honest about everything. The boundaries of their relationship are negotiated and renegotiated. They check in with each other. They talk. They are best friends. This is more than I see from a lot of monogamous couples I know.

There are, like, ten zillion ways to have a relationship, and not a single one is better than any other. Think about what you want and do whatever the hell that is. Make sure everyone in the relationship is on board and feeling happy and jazzed up. Communicate, communicate, communicate. If you're communicating, no one is betraying. We only betray when we aren't feeling heard or don't think we have the ability to be heard.

When I got out of my last relationship I questioned my once staunch views on monogamy. I wasn't sure if it would suit me in this new mode of life. Eventually, I realized monogamy was my jam. When I met my husband, I knew I just wanted to be with him. But, do we really know if this is the way things will always be? Perhaps we'll want to bring a third person in to join us in life or have a threesome or a foursome or a gang bang. Who knows? We want different things at different phases of our lives. Not all the time, but sometimes this happens. There is nothing inherently better or worse about any type of relationship. There is nothing wrong with relationships that don't fit strictly into a poly, open, or monogamous mold. Much like sexuality, relationship styles are fluid and should have the room to change and shift depending on a variety of factors.

The key thing here is honesty, trust, and communication. There is no betrayal. Cheating is betrayal. Cheating is lying.

If it's part of your primary relationship agreement to have other relationships, emotional or physical, and you've discussed it beforehand, it's not cheating. Having a healthy, stable relationship means sitting the fuck down and talking about it.

At the heart of it, cheating is about respect for the person(s) you're in a relationship with. If you don't respect someone(s) enough not to cheat on them, you should dip.

Sex therapist Dr. Dulcinea Pitagora puts it perfectly: "The difference between cheating and open relationships is consent from all parties."

It's about talking about it beforehand and figuring out what you're comfortable with. Even if the open policy that works for you doesn't involve talking about the other relationships you have, if you choose a "don't ask, don't tell" policy, you've still agreed upon that policy beforehand. If you don't want to hear about it because it makes you feel shitty and/or jealous, that's fine if you're fine with that kind of relationship. As my friend Malgosia once said to me, "Awesome things will happen if you choose not to be a miserable cow." Word up.

WHAT IT TAKES TO MAKE BOTH MONOGAMY AND NONMONOGAMY WORK

The truth is, a lot of people want to be okay with non-monogamous relationships and can't. I'm not over here telling you monogamy is dead and everyone should have sex with each other. It's okay to be monogamous if that's what you want. It's okay to do whatever works for you. It stops being chill when you're in a relationship—whatever relationship—that doesn't work for you.

No matter the relationship, it takes being able to communicate thoroughly. That is the bottom line.

Dr. Pitagora says there needs to be a willingness to take a risk and say something that may stick in your partner's mind (or yours) forever. You have to be willing to make things awkward. You have to trust your partner enough and have enough confidence in them to be able to have those conversations. You shouldn't have to worry that you "can't take something back" if you're voicing your desires or curiosities. If they judge you for all eternity, constantly bringing up the time you asked what they thought about a period of sexual openness in your relationship, there is something deeper going on there. If they shit a brick because you suggested giving monogamy a try, that's saying something about a dissonance in communication. You need to be able to have conversations that you can see through without getting antagonistic. You need to be willing to tolerate the discomfort of unfamiliar conversations. You have to be open to listening.

You need to make sure you have what you need from the relationship. You need to ask yourself if you have everything you want and are comfortable with what is or is not happening with other people.

If there is jealousy, anger, and feelings of betrayal, it may not even have to do with the physical sex that is happening outside of the relationship. Jealousy is a natural human emotion. Be able to recognize its roots. They might not be where you think. Most of the time, it's about what's happening inside the relationship itself. The angry feelings are linked to a lack of communication and respect for each other. Without the communication, you can't make things work.

Don't try to shove yourself into this crappy box of white-picket-fence conformity just because the world says you should. The kicker? A lot of understandings about your relationship and what works within it are going to change as you grow together. You also need to be flexible in how you figure things out. Dr. Pitagora says that people come to her wanting some kind of relationship structure but aren't sure what it is. There are so many different relationship styles. People have to be willing to start from scratch and figure out what works for them. Every relationship is a unique, individual thing. It has to be created and customized by the people involved. You can call it whatever you want to: poly, monogamous, monogamy-ish, open, closed when you're in the same city but flexible otherwise—whatever, but your version of that relationship will be different because you and your partner(s) are the only people who are creating that relationship.

Remember, cheating and discomfort in trying a new relationship style are not the same thing. Cheating is the end. You can't cheat on someone and then backtrack. You don't get to betray someone and then say you want an open relationship. Broken is broken, no matter how you look at it. Open is open, and it's kind of beautiful.

HOW TO MOVE ON FROM CHEATING

There are two people that have to move on from cheating—the cheater and person who's been cheated on. Here is how to move the hell on and find love that is worth your time.

Step 1: Forgive Yourself

For a cheater, it can take a long time to fix and move on from that behavior. I still have a lot of guilt about my past actions. I started writing about relationships as a sad way to confess to the internet all the terrible things I'd done (and to brag about all my slutty adventures, let's be real). Everything I'd done, all those fuckups, chipped away at my soul for a long time while I paraded fake confidence and a no-fucks-given attitude.

You have to remind yourself every day that things are going to be all right. I still feel like an imposter sometimes. You never get to a point of being perfectly okay. Some days are better than others. It isn't a fixed state of being. One day you'll feel like a fully formed human, and other days you'll feel like a flaming turd.

You may never feel like the person you were before all the cheating happened. I don't feel like the same girl. I probably won't feel like the same girl I am today five years from this moment. Every day is a learning process, and some days are better than others.

The dark moments are combated by a lot of self-motivation. When it comes to cheating, it isn't about self-restraint or controlling these dark impulses you have; it's about figuring out what's important to you and who is important to you. Figuring out your priorities makes you want to not do stupid things. The desire to ruin your own life becomes less pronounced.

For the person who's been cheated on, it's about recognizing that you aren't to blame for another person's actions. It's coming to terms with the fact that this shit happens. Sure, there were likely fucked-up things in the relationship that provoked your partner to cheat, so it's time to move on to something better. Look at your place in the situation and better yourself in the ways you can. We can always be better. Not every partner is going to cheat on you.

Recovering from cheating means knowing your worth, wanting more for yourself, and finding a love that sustains you—one that makes you feel whole.

Step 2: Do Some Shit That Makes You Happy

You know what is a great way to fuck yourself over after cheating? Wallowing in it. Instead of throwing yourself a pity party wherein you bathe in self-loathing, blame, and guilt, try throwing yourself into productive habits.

Partying may feel amazing while you're doing it, but it can wind up fucking you up if not handled responsibly. Become a better version of yourself. It's the ultimate "Fuck you" to the past and to anyone who's ever hurt you.

Redo your room. Build some furniture off Amazon Prime. I highly recommend a coatrack. It really did the trick for me. Go through all of those photos you meant to hang and never did. Get to nesting. Re-create a space that feels cozy and comfortable for the new stage of your life. You want to move forward making your life better.

You don't want to spend years thinking that the relationship was a waste of time and you learned nothing. Put the lessons of betrayal to use by becoming the stronger you you're meant to be.

DIY projects aren't the only way to self-improve, obviously. That is some basic-bitch-level shit to some. If you can't use a screwdriver for shit, throw yourself into your work or a passion project. You need to stay busy. The key to healing is staying busy. It's a lot of "fake it till you make it."

However, "busy" doesn't mean blocking out your emotions or feelings. It doesn't mean you're biding your time until the heartache subsides enough so that you push the shitty feelings down where you can't see them anymore. That's not healthy. "Busy" means expanding your life and deepening it to be better in whatever ways work for you. Choose things that make you feel better and stronger in the long run. I cheated and was cheated on. I decided to throw myself into my life in New York and network my ass off until I developed my writing career into something other than a WordPress blog in serious need of a grammar check.

Sometimes you're really just not fucking over it and need to do something to cope. Trade in two bottles of wine a night for activities that sustain you. Do shit that makes you feel good about yourself.

Step 3: Reacquaint Yourself with Love

Love isn't about guesswork. It isn't a game you play, one where you aren't sure how close you are to losing. Love doesn't make you feel lost or worried all the time. A real love is one that you can throw yourself into without a care in the world.

No one who loves themselves cheats. No one who loves themselves gets cheated on and stays. You may think you're on the high horse and nothing you do has consequences. It does. You're acting like a douchebag. It is an act of pseudo-empowerment, and that behavior is for fuckboys and fuckgirls, not kick-ass feminist leaders.

The only way to stop cheating is to discover and cultivate some self-worth. You do that by making yourself kick-ass without a partner. I flung myself into digital media from the bottom rung as an editorial assistant at a start-up. I stayed late most evenings to contribute articles to the site on everything from love to drinking to fitness. I focused on my career, and you know what? Eventually, I was noticed by my superiors. Before I knew it, I had a slot on the editorial calendar for weekly pieces. I believed I could do it, and I made it happen. I became the person I wanted to be. I refused to be in a relationship until someone worthy came my way. I knew I was a talented writer on the rise, a funny and charismatic person, and a loyal friend. I was no longer willing to date just anyone because I wanted to feel wanted. I wanted myself.

The only way to not get cheated on is to stop dating assholes. You're a lucky bitch, because I have plenty of shit to say about all of that, too, in the next chapter.

Step 4: Let Yourself Love Again

The first question I asked after my breakup with the abusive psycho was, "Will I ever find love again? Will anyone ever love me again?"

While these were genuine concerns, the answer is *fuck yes*. Fuck yes because you are awesome. It's easy to get bitter as fuck after being cheated on. How the hell can you trust anyone ever, right?

You cannot do this to yourself. You have to be willing to let

yourself love again. Be open to love. It's true that love has the ability to fuck you over. This is the way of the universe, but it doesn't
mean you close yourself off to it.

It's good to take a break from dating and spend some time
alone, but one day you have to get back out there and fall in love
again. Falling in love again is the way to forget all of the bullshit of
the past.

Of course, now that we've been super positive about letting
love in again, let's talk about how to let love go, even when you're
not ready to.

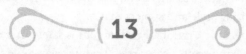

Breakups Are a Cunt

The woman you are becoming will cost you people, relation-
ships, spaces, material things. Choose her over everything.
—Unknown

I couldn't believe he was here standing in front of me, outside
of the gym, telling me he wasn't sure he could be what I needed.

It felt as if I were outside of my body, like a waking dream, the
kind you have where the details mirror your real life so exactly that
you can't tell if it's a dream at all. It didn't feel real. I'd feared something exactly like this in the dark recesses of my imagination, often
playing out these doomsday scenarios in a self-flagellating way for
months. I'd told myself the likelihood of this happening was probably zero and I was basically that meme where the cartoon rabbit is
in bed with crazy eyes and it reads, "Me not sleeping so I can imagine highly unlikely disastrous scenarios." But here it was in front of
me, actually taking place.

Here we were, in front of the gym on a Wednesday morning in
2017, on a dirty East Village sidewalk. My boyfriend told me he felt
like a burden and that he'd had two panic attacks in the last four
days over the possible invasions of privacy that were hanging over

us due to internet harassment and bad press connected to my provocative writing style and subject matter.

He had become irrationally afraid for his safety in months leading up to this moment. He worried that people would come after me (and him) in violent ways physically and online. He constantly imagined that our private information would be stolen or posted publicly, endangering us. Every time the trolls came, which they tend to do in packs, he would freak out. He was the only person on planet Earth that I needed to assure me that everything was all right, and he didn't. He made it worse. He made it about him and how my stalking affected his feelings.

As we stood facing each other on this warm September morning, he assured me it wasn't my issue, it was his issue.

He said we would talk about everything that night. He wasn't sure if he wanted to stay together or break up. He left me standing there, shaking and crying.

Just days earlier, we'd joked about how there were no two people in the world happier than we were. We joked about that a lot in our three years together. I'd been so full of hubris. I felt sorry for my single friends who hadn't found love like I had. *They'll understand what it's like to be really loved and treated like a queen once they find it. Every girl deserves this kind of intense, supportive, wonderful love.*

The love of my life, or the person I believed to be the love of my life, left me while I was writing the first draft of this book—he left me the day before I decided I should draft this chapter. I wrote most of this anecdote while sobbing and snotting into my bathrobe sleeve, shattered into a million pieces.

Three months before, he'd asked my father for my hand in marriage. He didn't know my dad told me. I told him I knew he'd asked a few hours after we stood outside the gym and he took the first grueling step toward ending the life we'd built together.

He'd asked my father to marry me. He was making plans to propose. And now, the love we shared was quickly evaporating.

After he left for a 10:30 meeting, I pleaded via text, "Nothing has changed for me. Please don't throw away the great love of your life. I would marry you tomorrow if you wanted to marry me tomorrow. Please don't throw away this love. Please."

Then through tears on the elliptical machine at New York Sports Club: "We were supposed to be a tree." It was something we used to say—that when we died at the ripe old age of ninety-eight, we'd be buried in the ground and planted as a tree.

I meant it. I would have married him that day. I would have gone down to city hall in my gym leggings and married him. He came back to the apartment that afternoon only because I begged him to come talk to me. He made me a smoothie. He got into our bed to hold me.

And then he told me he was leaving me.

I was on a plane back to Chicago at 8:00 the next morning, a move that would be permanent. In the blink of an eye, life as I knew it had ended forever.

We had been so crazy about each other for so many years. It was all so easy. It felt so good to know that the love aspect of my life was taken care of and I no longer needed to worry about it. I felt completely at ease. I felt safe. "My boyfriend isn't going anywhere. He's in this for life," I joked with friends and strangers. It made me bolder in my writing. I knew I could say anything I wanted without consequence. It's not like I had to worry about a Tinder date googling me.

Logically, I knew it takes two people to make a breakup happen, but in the immediate aftermath, I masochistically went through every wrong step and fumble. I looked at our relationship under a microscope, scrutinizing every wrong move we'd made; every wrong step he'd made followed by a wrong reaction from me; to every wrong step I'd made followed by a wrong reaction from him.

Again, logically, I know that nothing could have made the love last no matter what I'd done differently, but I thought if I wanted it desperately enough, maybe I could locate the moment that set us on a path from being so very in love to our relationship crumbling and lying at our feet in shambles.

In February of 2017, seven months before our life together ended, we were featured in a spread in *Time Out New York* for a podcast we'd started about relationships. It wasn't a particularly popular podcast. My friend worked at the magazine and recommended us for a story on New Yorkers' sex lives. A few weeks after it was published, my boyfriend got some unwanted attention at the start-up where he worked. Nothing major, just some jokes made by his CEO, a friend for many years.

The attention from this led him on a journey of wanting to pull himself completely out of the public eye.

A week after the feature, I was laid off from the website where I worked, and my freelance career took off seemingly overnight. What could have been a disaster turned into one of the best things that has ever happened to me professionally. I went from writing for an audience of somewhere around five hundred thousand people to millions and millions of people.

With that kind of widespread name placement comes internet trolls and harassment. I had been harassed for years, but it quickly became much worse than I'd ever experienced. My boyfriend just couldn't take it. He couldn't handle the pressure. I couldn't make him understand that it was too late for him to be anonymous. He said he regretted every time he'd agreed to be in an article, doing the podcast at all, and the time he wrote an internet love letter to me called, "What It's Like Dating a Sex Writer."

His words stung. It made me feel like he was ashamed of me for what I do for a living. His opinion was the only one that mattered to me. I didn't give a fuck about anyone else; I just wanted my partner to be proud of me.

I can honestly say I had done nothing but love him. I wanted to support him. I had seen him through leaving his company to start a business, to leaving the business to pursue full-time work again, to the idea of moving away from New York. It was scary, but I knew that it was my job as a girlfriend and his support system to be there for him when he needed me.

His cowardice and anxiety over the trolls took an enormous emotional toll on me.

The worst of the harassment came after the (now-infamous) informational *Teen Vogue* anal sex article I wrote. The release of the article ended in a magazine burning by some famous, crazed, racist YouTuber with a neo-Nazi husband, and many death threats. I did not feel supported online or in my home. My boyfriend was panicking about the unwanted publicity and possibility of violence and was wholly unsupportive of my feelings. I know he didn't mean to let me down; he just didn't have the chops to be who I needed him to be.

We tried to work through it. We did what we could to make it work for both of us. I'm not shy about my feelings. He knew how upset and disappointed I was by his behavior.

I made excuses for him. I made excuses for myself. I convinced myself we would make it through. Every time something happened to throw a wrench in our relationship (me posting a troll's email on social media, my mentioning something cute my boyfriend said in an Instagram comment), I'd fight to make it better and undo his anger. It was shitty because it felt like I could do nothing right. I was "asking for harassment" by doing things I perceived were needed (like posting troll comments to raise awareness) or cute (like posting about our relationship because it, um, existed). We'd get back to where we were, back on track to loving each other. I'd convince myself, naïvely, that we'd be okay. That this time everything was going to go back to the way it was and we could rebuild what was broken. I think he was overwhelmed by his lack of strength. I believe he wanted to be stronger, he wanted to be able to handle it, and the fact that he couldn't do it was scary and damaged his self-esteem.

Of course, it wasn't about internet trolls, though he never said it. It was really that he didn't love me anymore. He wasn't able to grasp that what he was blaming on anxiety over doxxing was actually anxiety over wanting to leave the relationship. He kept saying all the right things and telling me how in love he was; meanwhile, he didn't feel that way anymore. I'd be anxious, too. I'd have panic attacks, too.

I thought our love could conquer anything. But my love wasn't enough. That's what hurt the most, I think. Nothing had changed for me. I loved him the same way I had always loved him. I wanted to give birth to his children and squeeze their fat baby thighs. I wanted to hold his hand when he was eighty and having trouble walking.

The pain sliced into my lungs. It was like nothing I had ever felt in my life. To love someone so much, to trust them so completely, to adore them with every inch of your soul only to have that love taken away is like having a limb cut from your body. It's like a death.

What comes out of this story is a hard lesson about the realities of relationships and the uncontrollable, untethered nature of love. Now that I've been through every kind of breakup there is, I know how to guide you through one, too. I'm here for you.

BABE, LET'S TALK ABOUT LOVE

The Beatles told us that love is all you need, but that isn't true. That is a lie we've been fed. Love isn't always all you need. Love is just one component in a very complex system.

This is a frustrating reality. When love is in your life, it feels like the crux of your world. To lose that seemingly stable aspect of your existence is terrifying. When love is falling apart before your eyes, it can seem impossible to see this event as just one part of a long, beautiful, scary, heartbreaking, emotional, gorgeous life. It feels like everything is over when everything is changing. You want to control everything so desperately that, when you can't, it's enough to send you into a full-blown meltdown.

In the last toxic days of a relationship, you spend so much time believing that if you just love your partner enough and give all your love without condition, that will help you fix everything; somehow, you will conquer every challenge. Love has to be enough. You keep pouring your heart into it more and more until there is no more love you could give.

And even after all of that, it just isn't enough. I had started this project wanting to show women that they could have a love like mine, one that was healthy, vibrant, and worthy of them. To my great dismay, and later solemn understanding of life's truths, even that love can be taken away. Even deeper still, it's okay because it is meant to be.

The lesson is that heartache is a part of our journey, too. Everything I've written in this entire book is connected to heartbreak. Though sexual empowerment is the crux of your freedom, heartbreak has its place inside of that framework.

The truth is, babe, love doesn't always last no matter how much you want it to.

I know that everyone saying that "this is for the best" and "you dodged a bullet" only makes it worse, all good intentions aside. You definitely want to punch those people in the face (don't, though!). Want to hear the fucking kicker? All that shit turns out to be true, eventually, but only when you believe it yourself. You know how Adele basically said that she'd find someone just like her ex because he was a dime a dozen? You won't find someone like your ex. You don't want someone who is a dime a dozen.

Let me tell you why you are better off and how to get through this in a non-cunty way, as one woman to another. Because we have all been through some shit.

Let's get through the breakups, the disappointments, and the heartache like we get through everything else: like badasses.

ALLOW YOURSELF THE LEEWAY TO BE EMBARRASSING

I was so fucking embarrassing through this breakup, you guys. Seriously.

Don't fucking pretend you're not going to text your ex a bunch of embarrassing shit. This is a lethal mistake many people make. We tell ourselves that we're not going to text, we're not going to call; we're going to be strong. And guess fucking what? We break. Every single one of us texts our ex and calls them eighty times on a vulnerable night (both sober and after too many cocktails).

This leads us into that spiral of shame, the one we have after we get hammered and do stupid shit. Texting your ex is the stupid thing you did while drunk.

You've got to forgive yourself for this. Instead of setting up unrealistic parameters wherein you allow yourself no self-understanding about your own lack of control during intense emotional stress, just allow yourself to text your ex.

Listen, you went through some serious shit. I was in a relationship for multiple years. Those feelings of love and devotion don't just disappear because your partner turned out to be a total douchebag. You don't just get over it and suddenly become happy and great. Sorry, it doesn't matter how strong you are. You are a human being. You will oscillate between periods of intense sadness, tragically desperate love, and venomous anger.

Set a time limit for the messages, calls, emails, internet stalking, and whatever else. Give yourself a six- to ten-week time period wherein you can do whatever the fuck you want. Do you want to text your ex about something that reminded you of them and how much it hurts you, even though you know it gives them emotional power? Just do it. Let yourself do it.*

---

* Unless they have specifically asked you not to contact them. If this is the case, *do not* do it. You might find yourself looking down the backside of a restraining order if you do, girl. You are too fabulous for that! I mean it. Do not.

Get everything out. Get it all out there and say everything you need to say. Push it out of your system. Flush it out of your bloodstream. After a breakup, especially one we didn't plan or want, there is a ton of unfinished business and feelings.

Actual embarrassing things I sent to my ex* in the first few weeks after he broke my heart and left me without our future or a place to live:

September 15, 2017, 4:14 p.m.
It sucks when the person you used to tell everything to isn't there anymore.

September 16, 2017, 10:09 a.m.
I'm still in the phase where I start crying every time I realize you will never kiss me again or hold me or just lie next to me and laugh.

September 16, 2017, 10:49 a.m.
Every single day of my whole life, I didn't want to love like that because I thought that one day, out of nowhere, someone could stop loving me and without warning, life as I knew it would be over. I didn't want to be blindsided like that. But you made me believe that it wasn't true, that love really was available to me and everything would be OK because you loved me. And then it turned out to all be true.

Let yourself get the pain out there. It doesn't matter if they know

---

* And, no joke, there are probably over seventy-five thousand more just like this. I found these after fifteen seconds of scrolling through my messages.

they hurt you. They obviously hurt you. If you don't say the shit you need to say, you will be racked with guilt for much longer. You'll wonder if you had just said "that one thing" if everything could have been different. In the end, it will not matter, and it certainly does not make you weak.

On October 18, exactly six weeks after my breakup and the day before I turned twenty-seven, I blocked my ex from my phone, the last connection I had to him. He was already blocked on social media, his emails were spammed, and his GChat blocked. This was the very last string, the final lifeline. This was the end. I haven't spoken to him since, and I never will again.

After the six- to ten-week period, you must stop. And I don't just mean, "Okay. Done with that pishposh." You know, where you say that and then next week you send a three-hundred-word text about how sad you are and how you will always love them.

I mean, you have to stop. You must delete their number, block them on every social media platform, and send their emails to spam. You get your grace period. You give yourself blanket forgiveness, and then you get that person the fuck out of your life. Deal?

IF YOU CAN GET THE HELL
OUT OF TOWN, GO

I know for many people, it's not possible to pick up and leave after a breakup. Luckily for me, I had the privilege of being freelance and could peace the hell out to see my family the next day. I never put my name on our apartment's lease. I'd chalked it up to laziness, but perhaps I knew this was all impermanent somehow.

If you're not close with your family, go stay with your best friend. Get away from your ex. The only thing that helps heal heart-break is distance and time. If you can put distance between you and your old life, it is a cathartic relief. The night before I flew to Chicago, I asked my ex to go stay in a hotel. I slept with the light on, surrounded by our things, all symbols of the broken life I had cherished.

I woke up with a heart-wrenching gasp, thinking it was all a nightmare. I reached for my partner, but he wasn't there. It was all real. Getting home into my mom's arms was heaven. It lifted a weight off me. I took a hot bath and cried in my robe, surrounded by the people who loved me unconditionally—love I never had to question.

If you can get the fuck away, you must. There is always a way to leave. Do not stay with your ex. Do not do it. Even if you have to couch surf while you find a new apartment, you must not stay there. It is poison to your mental health. Run. Run the fuck away. Go.

CHANGE SOMETHING ABOUT YOURSELF THAT YOU'VE ALWAYS WANTED TO CHANGE

Three days after the breakup, I got a killer bob. It was the haircut I was always meant to have. I'd been wearing my hair nearly waist-length, mermaid-style for my entire life. My ex didn't want me to cut my hair. He was vehemently against it.

I walked into a salon I had never been to before. I met Charles, a genius who saved me. He called it the Freedom Haircut. He chopped my hair off. He gave me gorgeous bangs. He allowed me to emerge from the ashes of my old life as a sexy, smoldering diva ready for the next chapter of my new bomb life.

Do something fabulous. Get a new haircut, get a facial, get a massage, pierce your belly button, get a tattoo,* go skydiving, learn how to shoot a gun, buy a ticket to Paris.

Do something a little wild, something you've been scared to do but have secretly dreamed of doing. I don't mean go out and do drugs or be self-destructive. Have an adventure that pushes you outside of your comfort zone. Do something you know you'll love but that your ex would hate. Fuck your ex; they can suck it.

Make a promise to yourself: Never do anything for a partner ever again. Never hold yourself back for another person ever again.

I'm done changing myself to make other people happy. You should be, too. You are fucking fabulous, and anyone who would want to change you can get fucked by a giant black spiked dildo (and not in a good way).

MAKE AN AMAZING PLAYLIST

Make two different playlists—one full of kick-ass, empowering music and one full of sad songs about heartbreak and moving on. Kesha's "Rainbow" and everything by Tegan and Sara helped get me through my breakup. As always, "Linger" by the Cranberries carried me into the light in the darkest of times. RIP, Dolores.

Music helps to remind you that there are people out there feeling heartache, too. It reminds you that you are not alone. Matters of the heart are intense and overwhelming. It helps to feel less alone.

---

* Do this, or any permanent change, with caution. Like, maybe don't get SINGLE AND READY TO MINGLE tattooed to your lower back. I mean more along the lines of getting that dove on your shoulder that you've been putting off for two years.

Stay away from the songs, bands, or artists that remind you of your ex for a little while, but don't allow your ex to ruin your music. Create a playlist with some of your favorite songs, along with the ones that remind you of your ex. Slowly add those songs back into your life. This may take some time. It's a little like weaning yourself off the pain and back into a state of peace. Time has a way of fixing these things. The human mind and emotional palette are exceptionally resilient and are literally designed to be able to cope with heart-wrenching loss. Your body does not want you to suffer.

You may need to put on the sad playlist from time to time and lie in your bed and weep. That's okay.

CRY YOUR HEART OUT EVERY SINGLE CHANCE YOU GET

There will be good days, and there will be bad days. Grief is a process. All of that "five stages of grief" stuff is total festering dog shit. Some days you will amazing. You will be RiRi. Other days you will feel like crap. Some days you will barely think of your ex; other days you will be crippled by memories and sadness.

Do not stifle yourself with fake stoicism. You are not made of steel. Cry. Every goddamn chance you get. Let the emotions well in your eyes and catch in your throat. Lean into it, and let it overtake you. Cry until you have no more tears to cry. And then, cry some more.

You'll find you have more tears after all that, so cry again. Crying is a deeply healing, human thing. Never be sad or upset that you're crying. You will be, but try. Even if it has been weeks, months, or years since the breakup. To cry is not weakness; to bottle up emotions and fear vulnerability is weakness.

It's good to admit when you're not okay. In many ways, it's braver than pretending everything is just damn peachy. In 2013, I left a man who treated me very badly, the abusive one I cheated on all the time. I still was not okay even though it was my choice to end things and even though I didn't love him anymore. Recently, I found a note I'd jotted down in my phone during that time.

Today is a particularly bad day. I knew my alarm would go off at 7. I was awake by 6:20 at first feeling completely exhausted and then the creeping anxiety of being alone and without him came over me like it hasn't in the last two days, since the day I dropped his keys off with his doorman. I don't know if it's the lack of sleep, it couldn't be the 3 beers I had last night (I don't even like beer). Maybe it's profound regret. I don't know but today I am not okay. I know that it's okay to not be okay. Especially 3 days after a breakup but I am not okay. Those questions are on my mind again. Did I make a mistake? Did I let a truly wonderful man leave my life? Am I ever going to find someone? My heart is aching like I didn't know it could anymore. I know there were reasons, I wasn't truly in love with him anymore, which means that the breakup had to happen. I forced his hand, I made him call me and he made me do it. I keep hearing his broken voice in the back of my head. The crackling sobs that I'd never heard before. It makes my skin crawl and my stomach churn when I think about that phone call. I am not okay. I'm really not in the place yet where I can say, "I am not okay, but I will be." Right now I'm just not okay and not sure that I ever will be. It doesn't matter how many people I talk to or how many times my brother and best friend tell me that I made the right decision and that this will all be okay in time, I am not okay. Sitting in my apartment, my phone clock telling me it's almost time to go, with the early-morning sun peeking through the windows signaling a new day, a time of day I am so very familiar with—the time of day when my thoughts are weary and my heart aches most—I am not okay.*

Looking back, I can hardly remember those feelings. I don't remember being that upset. My heart healed and let go of the pain. This happens so our hearts can open up to new love. I wasn't okay then, but I am okay now. I wasn't okay when my latest ex became my ex, but I am now. Women have highly developed emotional quotients. Some of the most stereotypical female traits are the strongest of all. We can learn from our mistakes, feel our emotions, and embrace a great capacity to love and experience empathy.

Count the ability to cry freely and feel fully as one of your most cherished strengths. Grow, learn, cry, heal, love. The woman you are becoming needs the room to grieve the loss so that she may discover her true path to greatness. The woman you are becoming is trying to break through. Let her break through. Care for her with tenderness so that she may show you her epic strength.

DESTROY THE EVIDENCE

When I was twenty-three, I wrote a post on my first blog *Cigars and Jewelry* about how you have to destroy the evidence of your old relationship. This still holds true.

Carrie Bradshaw once said (after a breakup with Mr. Big) that you have to throw away the pictures where he looks sexy and you look happy. She was correct.

---

* I clearly love being melodramatic, and that's okay.

Again, give yourself a time limit. Give yourself six months or even a year to keep the framed photos, the strips from various photobooths, the kissing pictures on Facebook and Instagram. Avoid going on a rampage within the first two weeks of the breakup and throwing every photo away. This may feel cathartic in the moment, but it will wind up making you feel lonely and desolate. You will long for those photos and memories.

Instead, give yourself some time to look at them and cry. Give yourself permission to reminisce and feel heartsick. Look at the photos when you need to, but hide them out of sight the rest of the time. You can go back to them when you need to take a peek, but you shouldn't have them in plain view as a constant, stabbing reminder of the life that you no longer have.

Once you've traded in fewer days of tears for more days of peace and acceptance (this can take time and will vary from person to person)—destroy the evidence. Get rid of the gifts that remind you of your ex-partner. Throw away his or her old T-shirt, the one that smells like them, the one that used to give you comfort. Throw it in the trash. Have a bonfire if that feels like the right choice for you. Get rid of the tangible pieces of your past life. I chose to do a Wiccan purifying ritual. My siblings and I filled a basin with water, lit sage, and had a fire. We put our hands over each element and said, "By fire, I cleanse myself. By earth, I cleanse myself." It was kind of cheesy and also amazing. They really had my back. We all deserve that in our lives.

Two weeks later, I spent two hours crying my eyes out as I deleted the hundreds of photos left on my computer that commemorated three years of happiness, one by one. I looked so happy, so content, so in love. It hurt so badly. It needed to be done.

You may still have moments tinged with longing, but without the evidence, it begins to fade into a distant memory. Time has power, by design by the universe, to soothe even the greatest heartache. Pain has no memory.

DO NOT TAKE YOUR FUCKING EX BACK

Don't romanticize your relationship for the rest of your damn life. You can do this during your grieving period. You totally can. All you want. You can wallow in the love lost and even blame yourself if you'd like. Whatever. You need to immerse entirely in the pain that is awash. Just remind yourself of the bullshit. This person was a little bitch who couldn't be the man or woman you deserve.

You cannot make someone want to be with you. You cannot make someone love you, and you shouldn't have to. For fuck's sake. That is bare fucking minimum. Love should be a given, not something you struggle to feel or receive.

Think about it. Even if my boyfriend had come back to me and told me everything had been a mistake and he was going to try to be the person I needed him to be, that he didn't want to break up, how would I have ever trusted him again?

It's the same kind of damage done that comes with cheating. There is something inherently broken. I would always know that he was capable of doing this to me. I would always know that he was so weak that internet trolls (internet trolls that weren't even his trolls) became a source of panic for him. I would always wait for him to leave me. I would be walking on eggshells for the rest of my life, waiting for some tweet or email to send him into an emotional tailspin.

No, the damage had been done. The damage has been done for

you, too. Even if they come back and want to work things out, even though all you want is to forgive him or her and make it work, don't. Just don't do it.

Even if it makes you collapse in dismal, gut-wrenching suffering to walk away, you've got to. Walk away. Just walk away.

There is nothing to save after this shit has happened. Do not ignore reality.

If your partner shows you who he or she really is, believe them. If they show you what they're capable of, you know more about them than you ever did before. Internalize that lesson to make you stronger. They are not worthy of you. They are a fucking coward.

ACKNOWLEDGE THAT YOUR EX HAS CHANGED INTO SOMEONE ELSE, AND SO HAVE YOU

In relationships, you need to mesh on life stages, and expectations, and goals, and your ability to be supportive of the other person when one is struggling or one is succeeding tremendously. This meshing is part of that complex system that includes the love that you were told was the only thing you needed.

You have to accept that people do change. Sometimes you change with your partner; you help them grow and they help you grow. When it's the right match, you grow together forever until you're old and wrinkly and literally start shrinking.

Other times, individual growth doesn't lead you to the same place. It can push your relationship apart and form a chasm between the two of you. If both of you don't work tirelessly to fix the gap, there is no chance of its being bridged. If only one of you wants to mend the break, it won't get fixed. Even in times when both of you do try to make it work, it still doesn't work every time. There are a million micro-scenarios in which a vast array of small micro-occurrences leave you with a breakup and a broken heart.

My ex-boyfriend was once totally into being a part of my work. He served as the subject of many articles. I turned my hands into vibrators for a story, and he was a willing subject. I got a boyfriend pillow and dated it for a few weeks. He was all about it and gave me some choice sound bites.

Then he changed.

First, he didn't want his name in any pieces, then he wanted the podcast taken off iTunes, then he didn't want me to talk about my relationship in any capacity.* He changed, and his priorities shifted. He became obsessed with having a private life. It didn't matter how many times I tried to explain that the ship had sailed and the internet is forever and can never be erased because he just didn't see it that way.

I grew away from him. My career continued on an uphill trajectory. I got a book deal. There were minor talks of a reality show with me and some of the women in my industry. Things were popping off for me while he was headed inside of himself.

He wanted a house in the suburbs with a simple job and life (his words), while I wanted to explore the reaches of my influence and create work that started a dialogue and changed attitudes around sex. He saw my ambitions as something at odds with his desired future. As long as I was getting "famous," his privacy was threat-

---

* We had a huge fight about the stories where he's mentioned in this book only a few days before the gym-robe-snotting incident. I don't use his name, as you've probably noticed, but that didn't matter in his mind. He was not having it.

ened. It served as a catalyst to a later loss of desire to fight for what we had together.

My vision departed from his. I wanted to be his wife and have his babies. I wanted to do it all. He couldn't separate the growing popularity from our relationship. It was too much for him. I wanted to fix the gap growing between us; he didn't.

Breakup and heartbreak.

If you change, if you grow, if you start to be your best self and move forward in your life, pay attention to your partner. Help him or her grow with you. Be accepting. Have empathy. But be realistic. You cannot grab them by the feet and drag them with you if they are unwilling to grow and change with you. Everyone grows and changes in their own ways as they move through life, but if your person isn't in sync with you and grows away in their own direction, it's important to recognize this and let them go.

People can change, but they have to want to change. They can grow, but they have to want to grow. If you're following these lessons I've laid out for you and your partner or a potential partner isn't into it or doesn't straight-up encourage you, don't be with that person. You need a partner, not a festering limb you drag along for the ride.

Accepting that you cannot change people with your will is nearly an impossibility for human beings. We want to change people, but we can't. We want the people we love to love us and themselves, but they can't if they don't want to.

In life, we have to let go of things that don't nourish our souls. If your partner stops growing with you, leaving your soul in need of love and tending, you've got to trim it away and let it go. All of that shit people told you about being better off was right. I hate to say it when it hurts so fucking much, but it is true.

GET SOME ACTION

Don't rush into sex with someone else, but when you're ready, go out and get some action. Set up comfortable, easy, and trusting relationships with people you enjoy fucking. Let yourself heal. Spend some quality time with your vibrator, and then go find someone chill to fuck.

For some ladies, it's hard not to get emotionally attached when sex becomes a part of the equation, so if you feel you can't just go out and get some ass without becoming a hot mess—skip it.

If you can handle it, set up a dick/pussy date with someone from your past (not another ex) who you know is chill and good in bed. The second option is finding someone on Tinder or different app. I prefer option one because you know the person well enough to decide if they are a piece of shit or not. You don't want to fuck a piece of shit.

Also remember that even when you're fucking someone and aren't looking for love, that doesn't mean you shouldn't have high standards for the way this person treats you. He or she must treat you respectfully. You should be treated like a fucking human being and expect nothing less. If that person doesn't text you back, go fuck someone else. Casual sex is easy.

Respect in this case doesn't mean paying for food or taking you out on dates (it's a sex thing, remember), but this person should be texting you back. No booty calls at 2:00 a.m. That is rude AF. If this person makes you feel shitty about yourself, don't have sex with them ever again. Don't waste your time on anyone who is a waste of time. There will be moments when you feel so lonely, so vulnerable, that the thought of any sort of validation from another human in any way will soothe you. It won't. It will only leave you feeling dirty and gross (and not in a good way!). Will it make you feel good to have some person say, "You know where your pants are, right? Thanks for coming by," after they were inside you three minutes prior? No. Probably not. When you're brokenhearted, you are dealing with gaping emotional wounds. You need to do things that heal them, not things that reopen them.

If you're going to fuck someone, set up boundaries. Communicate what you're looking for and stay within those parameters. It might be that you have sleepovers, it might be that they have sex with you and get the hell out of your apartment, it might be that you want them to pop over during the morning for an hour. Whatever it is, do it. If the person acts like a fucking asshole, don't fuck them again.

The thing that makes a new sex partner worth exploring is the need to wash off the stank-ass bullshit from your last relationship. Your ex already took so much from you. Don't let him or her take sex from you. Don't let him or her or them take pleasure from you. That's fucked up.

YOUR EX IS NOT THE LOVE OF YOUR LIFE

Moving on means reminding yourself every single fucking day that the relationship is over because it was unfixable. The relationship is over because you didn't belong together. You couldn't give each other what you needed to allow your love to thrive.

It took a lot of coping when I had to make my own coffee, and only had myself to look after, but that was a fuck of a lot better than wondering if there was going to be a cataclysmic fight that day, if I'd wind up despondent and tear-soaked because my boyfriend couldn't handle a mean tweet that wasn't even directed at him.

No matter what, I'd rather hold myself on my own than hold the weight of someone else's problems on top of me. You deserve fucking better. You deserve more. You are the love of your life. You're the only person who matters. Nothing is worth compromising who you are.

My ex felt like the love of my life. He wasn't. He was the love of one part of my life. He was what I needed at the time. Six months later, I met my husband. It turned out my ex was the stepping stone I needed to evolve into the person I am today with the love I've found.

The same is true of your ex. Your ex is not the great love you lost. He or she was the vessel you needed to become the person you needed to become. He or she helped you grow into this version of yourself, the one so strong that you now need something more. It hurts so much you can feel like you will die from the pain. But you won't. I promise you, baby. You will not die. You will walk away and see that you are capable of stomaching an astronomical amount of emotion and hurt.

This ex-partner helped you realize your capacity for love, your ability to open up and be vulnerable inside of your strength. It made you stronger to accept new love, greater love, into your life. What a thing to behold, my love.

He or she helped you define what you do and do not want from a future partner. Your tolerance for bullshit is nil, and your knowledge of love is elevated. Eventually, you will look back and see that this wasn't a waste of time at all. It was meant to happen. You'll thank your ex, weirdly enough, this human you loved so much and depended on for so much, for fucking up your relationship. They made you a better you.

It is time for the next fabulous phase of your future. You are ready for the rest of your dope-ass life.

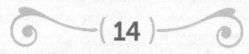

14

The Importance of Being Alone

Hey, girl. Can I talk to you for a second? Can we have a conversation between us sexy-ass ladies?

I have a question. I want you to really think about it, okay?

What the fuck are you doing in this dating game? What the actual tits are you looking for?

Love is dope, but let's be real—dating is a clusterfuck. It's an emotional time suck. It sucks life out of you faster than a day in the sun on a Colorado trail. It wears you out more thoroughly than multiple hours with your Magic Wand.

You want to find love, but you don't know how. Every relationship winds up being with some shithead with nine brain cells and an affinity for cocaine and ghosting. Even the long-term relationships wind up being toxic and passionless. That doesn't even take into account the people you date for a few weeks or months who wind up being a colossal waste of time. What the hell is happening here? Are we living in the fucking twilight zone? Tell me you know what I'm talking about.

Want to know why you keep fucking this up? It's simpler than it sounds and a lot harder to do than you'd think. You know, another clusterfuck.

It's because you have no fucking idea how to be alone. You don't know how to function without a love interest, a boyfriend or girl-friend, someone to flirt with, or at least someone waiting on the bench. You don't like being alone because you're scared. You're afraid of looking in the mirror. If you chilled the hell out and stopped journeying forth on this half-assed attempt at finding "the One," giving a chance to people who are covered in red flags like a rash, you'd have to look in the mirror and face the truth—you don't love yourself.

And guess what, Mama? You will never, ever find love until you do. You want to have a fulfilling life stacked with a fabulous partner(s) and wild, amazing sex? Get it the fuck together. Put down the pinot grigio and drop the iPhone. No! Don't you fucking text him. Hand me the phone, you stupid bitch.

Okay. Let's get to work.

A DEADLY GAME CALLED SERIAL MONOGAMY

One of my friends from college has a new boyfriend every two months. I am not exaggerating here. She will date one asshole, find another one, dump the current one, and move into a relationship with this other guy.

Or she gets out of a relationship, she says she's "single and ready to mingle," gets right the fuck back on Tinder, and has a new boy-friend a week later. She is never single for long. She'll tell me she isn't going to "apologize for getting out of a bad situation" and she "wishes people could be happy that she's found happiness again."

She says people are jealous that she always moves on so quickly. Now, this is probably true for some women. It's not easy for every woman to have a new partner lined up in a hot second. Though it sure is easier when your standards are nonexistent.

I wish I could say that her constant matching and unmatching is due to the fact that she's super amazing, hot, and funny (all of which she is), but it's not. It's because if a guy wants to date her, she's down. She will always do it no matter what. Hence the one-size-fits-all use of the word *asshole*. She once dated a gas station attendant who was white but wore cornrows and used the N-word. I wish I were joking, but alas, I am not.

The issue is that she feels shitty in whatever relationship she's in, so she goes off to find something else. She gets on dating apps and goes on dates with literally *anyone* who wants to be in a relationship without pause (doesn't matter who they are, what they do, or what they look like). If they want a girlfriend, she is down. Her criteria is as follows: *Do you want a girlfriend? Yes? I'm in.*

Serial monogamy is a half-assed, bullshit way to find love. If you wind up with a new boyfriend, girlfriend, or partner every few months, that isn't good. It means you have shitty taste. It means you're looking to find someone to complete you, when what you need is to complete yourself. You're looking for a missing piece that you will never find because the missing piece cannot be set in place by another human.

I have an honorary Ph.D. in being a fucking idiot. I've done both the single thing and the serial dating thing. It wasn't until I was single for almost two years that I figured out how I was supposed to be treated (ahem, like an absolute queen). I dated a bunch of jerks, one great girl I fucked over, and some more jerks—and was dicked around to the point where I was exhausted from the douchebaggery of it all. I then spent three years with the man I thought I'd marry, only to be back on my own again. And, weirdly, whole. Then, I spent more time alone. After that, my husband came along. All that time I was whole. I was growing, but I was whole.

All of this taught me everything I know about finding true love. Every single lesson.

When you are regularly looking for someone new, you don't learn shit. You stay busy to avoid doing the work internally. You can't stay out of relationships long enough to learn from past mistakes.

If you can't even bear to stand on your own two feet for any significant period of time, how can you expect to form a stable and equal partnership?

THE MYTH OF *"I JUST CAN'T STAY SINGLE"*

It's hard to tell when someone is being a stupid cunt and when they say they can't stay single. It is, in fact, hard to stay single when a) you have done a lot of work on yourself and have a stable life and a ton of confidence; and b) when you have done no work on yourself and keep dating every person you see.

The latter of which leads to the pile-of-shit relationships.

My friend with all the dickwad, under-accomplished, shithead boyfriends? Yeah, she's option B. Don't delude yourself into thinking that you're option A when you have no fucking reason on earth to think you're option A. You don't get to be option A because you decide you're option A. Look at your life. Look at your choices. You are not the motherfuckin' shit unless you have the motherfuckin' shit to back it up. And you don't have the motherfuckin' shit to back it up unless you have spent at least a few of your adult years 100 percent single. I'm not a time wizard, but I'd say at least two, preferably three to four.

If you have never done that, you are also option B. You don't hop from relationship to relationship because you "just can't seem to stay single." You hop from relationship to relationship because you don't know how to be single. You keep looking for love because you don't want to face the reality that is being alone. It scares the shit out of you.

If you wind up in a relationship a few weeks after dumping someone, you're probably fishing for it. You aren't being picky enough. You're not trying to be single. You're not doing any of that good-old soul-searching. You're jumping into talks with the next person who shows up. You clearly haven't got the standards up where they should be, girl. It's a pattern—a pattern that needs to be broken stat.

I get it—you might be so great that people just want to date you all the time, but that isn't an excuse. You don't have to date every single person who wants to date you. You shouldn't need that kind of validation. We think if someone shows interest in us, we should say yes and we should be so grateful to have secured that attention. Learn how to say no and wait for something that is truly worth your time.

I know I can't set precedents for life, but if I could cast a magic spell with my crystals and candles, I would make it so every person had to stay single for three months after a breakup. I'd make it a rule of life.

WHY BEING ALONE IS SO IMPORTANT

We're never taught that being alone is good. We're told that every-thing we do is about one end goal: marriage. It's that commodity model of female sexuality and worth, once again. Being alone isn't what we're supposed to want.

Our moms, dads, uncles, and grandparents feel badly for us if we're alone. We sit at the family dinner table, surrounded by people we hate-but-have-to-love-because-they're-family and are asked:

> *Why are you single?*
> *Are you dating anyone?*
> *What happened to that last boyfriend of yours?*
> *Don't you want to have children one day?*
> *You haven't been with anyone in quite a while. Are you okay?*

It's difficult to embrace your kick-ass self and enjoy your life as a badass single lady when everyone around you is constantly bom-barding you with the idea that you're unworthy if you don't have a partner in your life. Logically, you can tell yourself that you know they are idiots and don't know what they're talking about, but you have the creeping doubts in the back of your mind.

> *What if they're right?*
> *Am I pathetic?*
> *Is my career good enough?*
> *Is anything good enough if I don't have a partner?*
> *Am I worthless because no one is banging down my door right now to date me?*

None of that is true. Having time on your own is crucial to having success in a relationship later down the road. Many people can't manage a state of functional singledom. They view it as a defeat rather than a liberation. They are hounded and plagued by loneliness, and they are conditioned to feel it, despite how well everything else in their lives is going.

For many years, I jumped from crappy relationship to crappy relationship, or otherwise drowned myself in self-pity and alcohol (often both! Yippie!). I defined my worth by whether or not I had a partner. I didn't see myself as complete unless I could find love. It was unfulfilling and exhausting. I was dating people who treated me like shit and staying because I didn't think I deserved anything else. I didn't know there was anything else.

After a while, it became too much. I wanted more and didn't want to settle. Instead of jumping from boyfriend to boyfriend or girlfriend to girlfriend or hookup to hookup, I decided to completely cut dating from my life. For one year, I stayed completely single. I deleted my dating apps, stuck exclusively to one-night stands, and went on a journey of self-discovery.

I met a lot of interesting people from countries all over the world. I threw a bunch of wild parties at my apartment that had the neighbors ready to commit murder. I didn't go on any bad first dates. I didn't search for anything other than my future life. I started my first job at a company where I would eventually become a professional writer. I cut down on drinking (not a ton, but a little bit). I started journaling more than I had since I was in middle school and kept extensive notes on my hot, thirteen-year-old drama. I started to love being single. Like, really love it. I began making myself the person I wanted to be so that I could find a love that was nourishing to my soul. I made a list (yes, a real list) of all the mistakes I'd made in the past. I confronted my shitty taste in partners. I wrote out blog posts about being the other woman, cheating, and dealing with emotional and physical abuse. I owned my pain, and I owned my past. I stopped feeling ashamed of the broken parts of me and embraced every last ounce of the screwed-up things that made me the awesome weirdo freak I am. And you know what? I fell in love with myself. I fell so hard for myself that I worried about finding a partner lest I mess up the best relationship I'd ever been in. That is self-love.

Self-love is the baseline for finding true love. It is the foundation on which healthy relationships are built. We are fed these fairy tales of mountainous bullshit wherein we think we're these damsels in distress, waiting to be rescued by some white knight. We need someone else to make us whole. We're just waiting for love to complete us. This is nonsense. You have to be your own knight, and you have to save yourself.

You need to take a second to figure out what *you* want, not what you think you *should* want. All of this comes with time and patience. It comes with trial and error. It comes with figuring out what kind of life you can have on your own, the way you've chosen to build it. It is hard as all hell to stay out of the dating game. Dating is all anyone ever wants to talk about. The thing no one wants to tell you is that people will be jealous that you waited for the right person. It is so much better to be single than with someone who doesn't deserve you. It doesn't feel that way in the moment, but it really is the only way to find true happiness.

SINGLE AND READY TO
~~MINGLE~~ KICK SOME ASS

We've got to flip the script on singleness. We have to embrace it for everything it brings us. While there are certainly men who are berated by their friends and loved ones for their "singleness," the gender disparity is undeniable. Many studies have shown that men want love as much as their female counterparts (excuse the gender normativity here), but that doesn't negate the spinster/bachelor dichotomy. For most guys, being single isn't this sad state of being. A single guy is a bachelor; he is cool and fun. But a single woman is a hag; she's unlovable or broken. She's doing something wrong.

Imagine we stopped slut-shaming and single-shaming and just embraced this multifaceted, fucked-up thing we call being an adult human in the world? I mean, love is great, but have you tried loving yourself? It's way better.

What if all of that past single slutting around *actually* does help you figure out what you actually like in bed and what you want out of life?

Think about it, bitch. You can't learn about your body without sexual experience. If you are wild in the sack, it's probably because you already tried a bunch of fucked-up sex things you didn't like over the years. You weeded out the sex positions, toys, and orifices that you wanted nothing to do with long ago. I found out life is always better with a vibrator (solo and coupled), and while anal is not really my thing (all the time), I can always go for giving a prostate massage. I learned that a couples' vibrator is better in missionary, where there is bodily pressure, and I'd rather be spanked than choked. I wouldn't give up my hoeing days for the world. I look upon them with such fondness. I look forward to those to come with relish.

There were plenty of awful lays in my past, but I still wouldn't take a single one back, even if I do feel gross and weird about some of them. I know what I like, and I'm not afraid to ask for it. When you go into a monogamous relationship with assloads of experience, you know how to keep things interesting. You know what is good, what is bad, and what needs work. You're not going to lie in bed like a dead fish, too afraid to reach down and rub your clitoris for fear of bruising an ego.

We get confused and our vision becomes blurry when we're in a romantic relationship. We miss what is right in front of our faces. Our hearts and emotions get involved, and suddenly we don't know what the fuck is happening. We have to see the bad shit to know that the shit is bad. We have to be treated well and have good sex to know that it is possible. And it takes being out of the relationship to even recognize all of this fucked-up shit. Love is blind because love is a douchebag. Just kidding, but also I'm not.

We've got to use what we know from the bad fucks to help us figure out bad love, ya hear? Once you've had enough sex, both good and bad, you'll be pretty fucking picky about what you are and are not willing to put up with. And your partner is in good hands. How would many of my exes have known they liked their balls massaged with a finger vibe if I hadn't known that was something some people enjoy? How would your girlfriend know she prefers her clit orbited over direct contact unless you'd eaten a lot of pussy? Being a slut is a fucking fabulous thing. Sluts are better girlfriends. Sluts are better people.

Embrace your beautiful, sexy self. Literally (not literally) fuck the haters. Fuck them. You're not doing it right if people aren't hating on you.

As Dr. Seuss says, "You've got to be odd to be number one."

Use your sex-goddess status to love yourself and stop dating complete pieces of shit. The shit-dating time in your life is over. It's canceled.

YOU GOTTA BE WHOLE

If you stop relying on anyone else to make you feel whole, you will be able to find someone worthy of your shine. Dope people flock to someone who is true to themselves and owns their shit. It's sexy to know you're awesome.

A partner will never be the person who makes you whole. You have to be a full, vivacious, well-rounded person on your own. A partner is just a bonus—a cherry on the sundae, the triple settings on a finger vibe. If you need a romantic interest in your life to feel complete, your ass is compensating. Don't play.

It took four months for my previous long-term partner to lock that shit down. We'd known each other for a few years but hadn't gotten serious. We were both in different places in our lives. We stayed in touch. Then one night, he came to a party at my apartment having decided I was going to be his girlfriend. I didn't know this, obviously. I would have been super creeped out.

He had grown a beard and was looking fine. We started hooking up on the regular. He wanted a relationship, but I didn't. The less I wanted a relationship, the more annoyed he became. It wasn't "hard to get," per se. I was happy being single and didn't want a relationship. I was doing my thing and enjoying every minute of my life.

I loved my friends. I loved my job. I loved my freedom. I made him prove to me that he was worth my time. He persisted. He didn't give up. He knew what he wanted and was willing to put in the work. Eventually, I realized he was someone I could see myself with. He was someone who would enrich my already wonderful life. I didn't need him, but I wanted him. I could live without him, but I didn't want to.

When the relationship ended, I was still fine. Oh well. Loving yourself is actually the simplest way to find romantic love because you don't have to do anything. If you love yourself and know what you're looking for, the right person will manifest. They just show up. If you give a fuck about yourself, waiting isn't hard. You're dating yourself, your whole beautiful glorious self, so you could never be bored. When my husband came along, it took a long while for me to accept settling down again. I was loving my life and my freedom. He hung in there. He stuck it out. I married him. Love yourself and romantic love can follow.

How to Be Single

1. Invest in your friendships.

Start by investing in relationships that don't fuck you up. Take value in your friendships.

Your friendships should never come second to a romantic interest. There is nothing shittier than a woman who serial dates and/or finds a boyfriend and falls off the face of the earth. That isn't being in love; that is being a cunt.

When I say "invest in your friends," I don't mean a bunch of fake-ass people who you can spend the time with between relationships. Don't even fucking think about doing that. The older you get, the more you realize everyone is awful and that you hate them. You realize everyone is the worst and that's okay. You don't have to keep them around. You just have to love yourself enough to trim the fat and find your people. Not everyone is going to be about you.

Instead of surrounding yourself with a few fair-weather party people, pick a handful of lifers and stick the fuck to them. You know the kind of friends I'm talking about. Ones who are as about themselves as you are about yourself; the kind that make you feel good about yourself and proud of your accomplishments; the friends that are amazed by you and believe in you even when you don't believe in yourself. Pick friends that lift you up when you're down, ones that won't let you date fucking tragic morons because they expect better for you.

Focus the energy you otherwise would on finding love into the people who love you unconditionally. Try giving a fuck about people who want the best for you no matter what, the people who stick behind you through thick and thin.

Stop giving a fuck about what other people expect of you and start expecting shit of yourself. You only have a finite number of fucks to give. Don't waste them on idiots.

2. Learn to be physically alone (and love your space).

Yes, easier said than done, but practice makes it easier. Give your middle finger to everything that doesn't serve you. Learn to love your space and the choices you make for yourself. When you're the only one you need to please, everything can fall into place. The best version of yourself can find herself. Here are some ideas on how to slough off everything that does not serve you, the badass that you are:

1. Wear whatever you want. Buy things that make you feel sexy.
2. Take yourself out to dinner with a good book. Authors make wonderful dates. Plus, you'll learn to be comfortable in crowded places with only your thoughts to keep you company.
3. Go for long walks in neighborhoods you've never explored. Daydream about your future apartment or house.
4. Get a manicure. You have to put your phone down. You can't distract yourself with Instagram. You have to lean into the anxiety of being alone with your brain.
5. Make your room yours. Decorate it with relaxing salt lamps and fairy lights. Create a space that is only for you, one that has your style.
6. Take a new gym class. Don't bring a friend along as a crutch. Get your workout on and enjoy the sweat.
7. Find an online meditation and begin each day with it. It's only five minutes, and trust me, it gets you off on the right foot. Even before you've had coffee. We know that is saying something.
8. Take up the whole bed. Don't wait for some other person to "keep you warm." You cold? Get another blanket. A down blanket. A pink down blanket. Buy an enormous, memory foam mattress and sleep like a goddamn starfish.

Train yourself to love being alone. It takes practice, but you can do it. There is something so resplendent in knowing you need nothing but yourself to be happy. It is the ultimate peace of mind.

3. Shape the life you want. One you can do on your own with joy.

If you shape the life you want—the career, the apartment, the savings account—that's when you find a relationship worthy of you. You don't need a relationship with the person of your dreams; you are the dream. Your life should be a completely stable ship on its own sea of amazingness. Look at where you want to be in five years. I know a five-year plan sounds like some white-girl nonsense, but it helps you set realistic goals for a life that doesn't depend on other people.

1. If you have bad credit, get one of those credit cards where you put down a deposit. Basically, you give the bank a small amount of money ($300 or so) and then they give you a $300 credit limit. That way they're safe and you're safe. Pay the card off in full every month to build your credit. Eventually you can trade up for a real credit card!

2. Put away one hundred dollars a month into your savings account.

3. Don't buy boxed mac 'n' cheese for dinner every single night. Learn how to make nutritious meals. You don't have to spend a ton of money. Invest in a Crock-Pot and you can make enough food in one go for a whole week.

4. Add something new to your apartment every other month. It can be something small. Add a vintage

lamp from the flea market, a cool poster from Urban Outfitters, maybe have your dad send you that one quilt you've always loved from home. I found a millennial-pink tea set that shaped the whole theme for my apartment.

5. Stop settling in your career. If you are not in the job you want, start applying for the job you do want. If you don't have the credentials, start networking and building up relationships. Go back to school if you have to. If you want a raise, ask for the raise. Stop being fucking scared of risky choices that will help you get to where you want to be. In a few years, when you're in the job you want, obviously killing it, none of this will matter.

4. Revel in your badassery.

You are a motherfucking badass. Be the badass you know you are. Be her. She is *you*. Shut down those pesky, dehumanizing, "Why are you single?" questions.

Try these responses to those awful, pestering inquiries:

How about you ask about my job instead?
How about you worry about your own shortcomings?
My dowry is too high to tempt a husband or wife!
The GOP is ruling Congress; 'nough said. Why aren't you single?
I hate everyone; is that an okay reason?
I am perfect, so let me know when another perfect person comes
  along. Something tells me that is highly unlikely.

Shut them the fuck down, ma'am. Love yourself, you beautiful, sexy, smart, accomplished bitch! If you find that someone doesn't want to be with you because you have too much confidence, tell them to suck a bag of a zillion dicks.

Remind yourself every single day that you are the light of the world, baby. You are a person worthy of love and respect. You are kick-ass.

You are a fucking star. I'm not even just saying that, you sexy piece of ass. It's hard to believe that you are amazing when the world constantly tells you you're not. If you're confident, you're negatively branded as "too intense," "aggressive," or a bitch. If you tell it like it is, people don't know how to handle it. Don't fuck with those people. Those people are assholes.

You are fabulous. Work it. Live it. Now, go burn some sage to all your exes and move on with your sexy AF life.

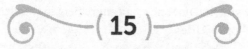

15

Getting a Partner You Actually Want

Prerequisite for all the people you date: He or she must be obsessed with you. No nonsense. No games. No ghosting. No lukewarm fuckery. Obsessed. If the person you're dating isn't balls-to-the-wall, head-over-heels obsessed with you, what is the fucking point?

Anything less is settling. It's not compromising, it's not being reasonable, it's staying in a relationship that is beneath you. And I don't know about you, but I'm tired of that being the expectation we have for relationships. That bar is low, and I'm not about it. I'm sick as shit of letting people get away with being dicks and cunts because we think that expecting more is asking too much. Nah.

You are an ever-changing, ever-growing human, but at the core of it, boo, you can't fuck with perfection. It's time to stand the fuck up and demand, expect, and achieve the relationship you want.

If you are loving the single life and have no interest in dating, don't date. Don't push yourself to have a relationship if you're into the way things are. If you want to do your own thing, do your own thing. If you want a relationship, make sure it's a fucking great one.

Self-love, self-love, self-love—check.

Getting a relationship you want means following a magic recipe. I can assure you that not one single ingredient in this delicious stew is "bullshit" or "excuses."

STEP 1: STOP ACCEPTING ASSHOLES

If someone is into you, there is no murkiness. There is no gray area. When it's right, there is no margin of error for doubt and crap. Stop settling for assholes who aren't over-the-fucking-moon into you. It is not worth your time. It is not worth one single, miniscule fuck.

If he or she is playing games, walk the fuck away. Are you sitting around wondering why a person sends you a Snapchat at the pool but never asks you to hang out? Are you feeling confused by the lack of reciprocation of oral sex, despite your giving it regularly? Guess what? Not that into you. Sure, some people may be *really* not into giving (or even receiving) oral sex, but if you ARE down to clown in Oral Town . . . are you going to stick with that person? Hm. Better not.

Have you dated people who said they weren't ready for labels? They just want to "take it slow and see where it goes"? Yeah, not that into you. Not worth a moment of your precious time. Not worth a single fuck.

We're so fucking scared of making a mistake, like we're going to miss out on some great person because we had a "no-bullshit" policy. We think if we wait around for a little bitch to grow up, they'll come around for us. Nope. Not a thing. There is no such thing as "the one that got away"; there is only the one that was meant to be in your life and proved it to you like a grown-ass motherfucker.

When we have little self-respect, born from a female legacy of being told we don't deserve it, we settle for douchebags. We are trained to believe that asking to be texted back, or taken on dates, or called someone's girlfriend, or treated like a priority is too much to ask. We don't want to be high maintenance or demanding. We have been trained to believe we're asking too much when we ask for the bare minimum. The truth is our expectations are sickeningly, embarrassingly, pathetically low. No wonder there is a fuckboy epidemic.

Asking for respect and to be treated like the rarest jewel in all the land is not asking too much; it's a fucking requirement.

You're not being demanding because you want to be treated like a human being. You're being a person with needs. If the person you're dating can't even be bothered to text you back, blows you off, disappears for days at a time, and then hits you up at 3:00 a.m. with an überclassy, "U up?"—that person is a fucking asshole. And you know what? Every single day you stay with that person is self-abuse. Every time you don't walk away from this shitty treatment, you are saying that you don't deserve better.

In my twenties, as a single lady, trolling for dick and dinner on Tinder and clubbing my face off (these two things are both unrelated *and* related, you know?), I used to date a lot of assholes. I've laid bare my soul in previous stories here. My dating life was a never-ending slew of assbags and losers who somehow also thought they were God's gift to mankind. I also dated my fair share of doormats: guys who just lay down and gave into my every whim. Suffice it to say, I've been on both sides of the asshole spectrum.

There can be only one asshole in the relationship, but there should be no assholes at all.

When my ex-partner—a person who is decidedly not a fuckboy—came along, I was ready for him and all the things he'd teach me in the following years. I'd been dicked around, and I'd done enough dicking around to have grown from it and decided I wasn't going to take that shit anymore. Empowered women don't date assholes. Women who love themselves love people who love themselves. We want partners who are fucking obsessed with us and treat us like queens—but who also don't take shit. That's the supreme difference between a woman with confidence and one without—the demand to be treated with respect and the intolerance for anything less.

You have to grow the hell up and decide you want a real relationship with a person who treats you like gold and is your best friend—and you have to believe you *deserve* that—and that's when it happens. Holding yourself to a high standard is how you wind up with a partner who is the gold standard. Self-love brings love, baby girl.

Boo. Sweet pea. Lover.

If you want a good relationship, ask for it. Don't wait around for someone to be nice to you. Lay out how this whole fucking thing is going down. If the person you're thinking of being with doesn't like these terms, fuck them. Ask for what you want and settle for nothing else.

Finally, don't beat yourself up for past mistakes. Learn from them. Use them to fuel the fire of self-growth. Don't get bogged down by the past; use the past as puzzle pieces to complete yourself. You are the beautiful patchwork quilt of every last fuckup, my queen. That is rad.

STEP 2: PICK A GOOD PERSON (FOR ONCE)

Ditch the assholes and pick a person who is nice. I'm not talking about that idiot tax attorney who says shit like, "I'm a really nice guy," on the first date. No. Red flag. Anyone who says they are "nice" is not nice.

Pick a good fucking person for once in your goddamn life. What constitutes a good person is subjective. It helps to make a list of what you like and what you don't like. Start with a list of all the people you've dated, liked, or loved. Categorize the good and bad character traits, the good and bad aspects of the relationship. It takes self-awareness to avoid being swept up into the cloud of lies of a player. Be aware.

FYI: It is not that hard to be a good partner. You just act like a normal human being. Feed the person you're dating, play with their hair, and text them back. It's respect. That is the key ingredient. And empathy. Respect for someone as a human being and empathy for how your actions make that person feel. Humanization in dating. Who knew?

Pick someone who is kind. This does not mean boring. *Kind* does not mean lifeless. It doesn't mean damp. It means choosing someone who actually treats you well. Someone who gives a fuck about you.

Kind does not mean dating a doormat. You want a confident, down-to-earth person who actually has their shit together. Someone confident enough to put you in your place when you're being a dick. Someone who understands you and loves you but who isn't afraid of you.

You want a person who is the wind beneath your wings.

Be ready for someone who is going to be kind to you and make you feel good about yourself. Be ready for someone who is going to make it all easy. It takes truly wanting it. You can't just declare that you're not giving in to dickwads anymore. You have to recalibrate what you're attracted to. If you have self-love, this will develop on its own. Be open to it.

Be on the lookout for red flags. Red flags include but are not limited to: not texting you back; referring to an ex as "crazy"; staying best friends with an ex;* always being on his or her phone; breaking plans; not having much in the way of a career; living off his or her parents; not liking physical touch; not introducing you to his or her friends; not paying for a single fucking thing; complaining when you ask him or her to spend quality time with you; referring to Holden Caulfield as a relatable character—unironically; thinking Bitcoin is cool—again, unironically; and so on. If any of these egregious red flags pop up during any dating or sexual encounter, do not give this person a second chance to be more of an off-color creeper. They are not for you. They do not deserve a chance when you know in the pit of your stomach that something ain't right. They do not have a right to your time. No one has a right to your time. If it doesn't feel good or right or like there are sparks, go grab a drink with your bestie after the date and lose that stranger's number. You are obligated to nothing. Ever.

Don't even play because we both know you've dated plenty of cuntrags. If you're a slutty, sexually empowered woman in your heart and soul, you've probably been through the shit. You've dealt with enough douchebags (I blame you, Tinder!) to know what you *aren't* looking for. Once you get fucked over by the wrong kind of people enough, you stop wanting to date playboys/girls/people and you *finally* choose the good person.

---

* Jury is still out on this one, but this is sketchy as fuck. If they are a courteous acquaintance, that is acceptable. We intermingle friend-groups. It happens. It is probably better than hatred, right?

No more twats who are just looking to hit it and quit it (unless you, too, are looking to hit it and quit it because, hey, a girl has got needs). No more immature shitpiles who ghost like it's second nature. It isn't sexy to wonder if someone loves you. Eventually, that player nonsense stops ruffling the butterflies in your stomach, and instead, it bores you. You want more out of someone and stop being afraid to demand it. Being alone is better than being treated like nothing. You want someone who treats you like a queen, their best friend, a valued person in their life deserving of respect. The weirdest thing happens when you decide you want to date someone who treats you well—you find someone who treats you well. It feels like some secret code, but it isn't. It's just the way it is.

There is so much beauty in living a strong, independent life as a nasty woman. You figure out what you want in the future because you've seen (and fucked) all the wrong people already. Somewhere down the line, after years of fuckery, you begin to wonder what it's like to be the priority. This is where you begin. You decide you want to be the priority in a person's life, and then you stop settling for anything less than this bare minimum. This ponderance of your own place in a relationship gives way to self-preservation and a desire for that something more.

Dating pigheaded, aggressive, pseudo-charismatic, cavalier alpha (if you want to even call it alpha) jock fuckboys or fuckgirls is the kiss of death for an alpha woman. It is the kryptonite to your success. If anyone dares to pull that crap, you show them the door. You have bigger proverbial fish to fry. You need someone who lifts you up to make you a better, stronger you, not someone who holds you back in a gray area of second-guessing.

Enough of the emotionally turbulent, passionate dillholes. You need to pick someone who brings you the fuck down to earth. When he or she wants to hang out with you, he or she does. It stops being weird that they respond to your texts all the time because they're obsessed with you. They should be. This person will be excited for you to meet his or her mom and to tell his or her friends about you. They will make plans and stick to them. They will have their shit together and want someone who wants to share a life. This person should want to be with you, do thoughtful things for you, and make you feel safe and secure every single day. There is no confusion because confusion only exists when it isn't right and your heart isn't in the right place. No doubts exist when it's all easy, adult, and normal. You know Stevie Nicks said that players only love you when they're playing. Stevie knows.

You should never have to worry whether or not they love you because they will make sure you know. When someone shows you who they are, believe them. When someone gives a shit, it isn't a game. They give a shit.

For many of us, it takes a long time to find this kind of relationship. You can say you want to find a nice person all you want, but you won't until you truly believe you are worthy of that kind of love.

STEP 3: BE SOMEONE YOU WANT TO DATE

You want to find someone awesome? You need to be a person you would want to date.

You do not need to change yourself if you're happy with your life. If you're happy being single, drinking, and raging, good for you. As long as your behavior isn't affecting those you love or your ability to care for yourself, you're entitled to live your life however you want.

Check in with the people around you. Listen to the people who want you to be the best you that you can be. Take time to look internally and ask yourself, *Am I happy? Is this the life I want?*

If it is, go forth and do you. The answer may not always be yes, but as long as it is, you're doing all right, babe.

But consider this: If you wouldn't want to date a person who's doing the same shit you're doing, it might be time to reassess your priorities.

When I was a hot-mess party girl, I figured people should just want to date me. I wanted a stable, sexy, smart, and sweet guy or lady who would be an excellent partner. I wanted someone who had their shit together when I didn't have mine together in any capacity.

An interesting, normal person was not going to date me. I was a disaster. I sure as hell wouldn't date someone who was as sloppy and self-centered as I once was. So why would they want to date me?

If you find someone you vibe with, you'd better make yourself someone he or she wants to date, and he or she had better do the same. Complaining about being single all the time, while continuing to be a Blackout Barbie, is not going to fix everything.

This shit takes work. You can't just sit up one day and say, "I'm the best version of me now. Here we go. La-la-la." That's not how it works. Self-love doesn't mean accepting all of your crappy, rude, bad behavior. It means growing and learning. Do not mistake the path to self-love and confidence for the divine right to be a douche. Want more for yourself, from the person you love most—you.

Self-love requires the ability to constantly improve yourself. Love the hot mess you are, and love the grown-ass woman you will become. Love her and nurture her every step of the way.

Start by doing small things. Cook healthy meals. Go to the gym to get your endorphins up. Limit alcohol consumption to the weekends. Work on a side hustle. You should always have a project outside of your full-time job, even if you think you're too tired to handle it. You can. Don't just sit there. Do shit to improve yourself.

Remember all the stupid things you did while drunk? If you've learned from those mistakes and are taking those lessons with you into your life, you're on the right path.

If you're going to change, change because you want to. If you're a train wreck, stop being a train wreck, because you want to remember what you did at least five of the seven nights in a week. Get it together, because you have goals and want to achieve them.

If you're going to make changes in your life, they have to stem from a place of self-awareness. The decision has to come from the desire to make your life happier and more balanced. If your choices are making you miserable, you have to think about what you can do to stop making yourself miserable.

If you want to find love, you have to be a person who is ready for love. If you come to a place in your life where you decide you're ready for a stable, healthy relationship, you have to look inward first.

Be willing to grow and change every single day. Evolve.

In the early days of my last (pre-husband) relationship, when I was still a blackout drinker, my partner took me to a comedy show. I don't actually remember much of the night, but apparently I got so blacked out that I was screaming at the talent onstage. We were thrown out of the club. This is just one of an unquantifiable number of times I did shit like this. I was so out of control that I had to stop drinking altogether, save for very special occasions, for two full years. I recognized these experiences were not the best representation of who I am as a person. Sometimes I still get embarrassed about them, but every single bad choice I made forced me to become more resilient and showed me what I was capable of once I stopped drinking all the time. When you have a fucked-up past, you wind up with an attuned sense of empathy for others.

Create rituals to help you heal. Traditional therapy is an excellent way to talk and work through your past mistakes, but you can do more holistic things as well. You can take the power into your own hands. Tuning into yourself and your needs is a daily practice.

Whatever the ritual is should feel cleansing. No way is better than any other—unless your way of cleansing past mistakes is to go out and make more of them. Don't do that.

I stick to a routine that involves a ton of physical exercise and taking immaculate care of my skin. I only have one body, and I love taking care of it. It makes me feel together and centered.

I write in my journal or I write incredibly revealing articles on the internet. It's a cathartic process and helps me move past my own mistakes. When someone who has had similar experiences reaches out to share their story with me, I feel less alone and they feel less alone.

You can write down your mistakes, fear, worries, traumas, or regrets. Make a list and read it out loud, and then tear it up and bury it in your garden. You can burn the pieces, if you feel like that would be cleansing. You can light candles and whisper your transgressions to the universe.

Your ritual can be less witchy or granola, if you want. You can call your best friend and outline everything you've done that makes you feel shitty. She will make you feel less alone. That's what she's there for.

Just don't live with the bad feelings and let them fester inside you. I've often thought I deserved to live with my mistakes forever and let them eat away at me. This suffering doesn't help you learn. Get those feelings out of you in any way you can and let them go. Forgive yourself.

When you've gone through shit and are in the volatile process of healing, you are offered the opportunity to see how the person you want to spend your life with deals with your pain. Healing is not an easy process. It is not easy. How they handle your self-care either brings fortitude and durability to the relationship or breaks it. Any love worth having can take the heat of an unencumbered anxiety attack here or there. Being able to love someone unconditionally as a whole, flawed, ruthlessly fucked-up person is the only love you should allow into your life.

STEP 4: SEE THE BIGGER PICTURE

Gain some fucking perspective. In times of self-doubt, instead of choosing to focus on my behavior that night at the comedy club, I choose to look at the person I've become. I choose to think about how my partner chose to take care of me that night. Though we've since parted ways and moved on to very different paths in our lives, he didn't leave me or make me feel like a piece of shit. He accepted my apology, and we moved on. We saw each other through a multitude of highs and lows. We approached our relationship and each other with love and understanding rather than hostility. Eventually, the love faded and we both moved on. That doesn't mean we didn't grow together and learn a ton about life. My marriage isn't always rainbows and sunshine up the ass. It takes work. But my husband and I are in this together and recognize that responsibility to each other.

I don't apologize for things that have happened to me in the past any longer. I don't apologize for things I could or could not control anymore. They are just a part of the batshit-crazy process of growing up and becoming a woman. It isn't until you become a real grown-ass lady that you find a love that lasts. I've found forever-love, one that is worthy of me. I have no doubts anymore. I'm the best. And I know in my bones that you will find love like that, too. You just have to be open to it.

Whatever your stories are—whatever the fuckups—they are a part of you, and that is a good thing. Once you're finished being a wild single lady, you can grab relationships with the same ferocity as you did your single life.

Self-love isn't about just accepting yourself as you continue to make a mess of your life under the guise of feminist ideology. You can do wrong. You are not infallible. You're fucking awesome, but you should be willing to shift aspects of your life. That's what real strength of character is—an ability to recognize the parts of your life where you could improve and being willing to make those adjustments.

You know what you get when you take two dope humans who

know what they want, are confident and full of self-love, give a fuck about their careers, families, and lives, and then put those two people together? A fucking power couple.

Kick-ass feminists make the choice to be in relationships that are worthy of us. Allowing yourself to emotionally invest in a person is the most sacred and beautiful thing a person can experience. Why the hell would you ever deny yourself love that is worth it?

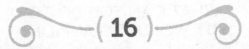

It Takes More Than a Book to Be Okay, but Knowing You're Not Alone Helps

As you've moved through the pages of this book, taken in the lessons, and thought about how they apply to your own life, I hope you've felt less alone. If you take anything from these chapters, my goal would be to leave you with that. Why? Because there is nothing worse than feeling alone. There is nothing sadder than feeling lost in the world and unsure of how to proceed in your own skin.

I'm not expecting you to be a different person after reading my book. I mean, fuck, it takes a lot more than a few hundred pages to come into your own. Having the resources available helps. Even after reading this book, and putting the lessons to work, things will be hard and there will be challenges all over. You're still you, but maybe a little bit stronger, a little bit readier to go out into the world and be your bad self.

One book isn't going to change the way you feel about yourself, but it can help. I'm here for you. I really am. I've been you. I'm still you. You're not always going to be sure of yourself, and you're not always going to feel like a badass bitch.

WHAT CAN YOU DO TO
PUT WORDS TO ACTION?

There will be times when you can't stand up for yourself. There
will be times when you're afraid. There will be times when you
feel like the ugliest, stupidest, weirdest person in the world.

Just remember that you are not alone, and we all feel that way.
That girl next to you on the subway with the fierce pink, faux fur
coat? She's felt that way. The girl at the supermarket who manages
not to put any chips or ice cream in her cart? She's felt that way.

Talk to people. Don't just hide in the shadows of your self-doubt
and cry into your TJ Maxx pillowcase. Tell your friends how you're
feeling. Share your stories. Remember that we are stronger together. We are killer. If we talk to each other and share the things
we've learned, we open up a new set of standards for the world
we live in. Once women start sharing sexting tips, and advice to
stop sexual harassers, and where to get the best leather harnesses,
these discussions become normalized. So talk about it. Talk about
it every single day. Face your embarrassment around sex enough to
talk about it.

You shouldn't put pressure on yourself to be a fully changed
woman and suddenly you're supposed to be fearless. You don't have
to do everything you've read about in this book. You can do some
of it. You can do it in baby steps or chapter by chapter. Maybe only a
few of the lessons stick with you. That's okay. But don't do nothing.

What makes you different is a willingness to make changes to be
your best self. That's the best we can do—be willing and start taking small steps to be our best selves. Finding love is an afterthought.
The real goal is loving yourself and trusting yourself enough to take

actions. I know it doesn't feel like it when all of your friends are off finding boyfriends or girlfriends, getting married, and having kids—seemingly without effort. But you don't actually need love to be happy. You don't. You've been conditioned to believe you do, but you do not. You need yourself and that's it. You are the only person who is going to be there in the end. If you don't love yourself and take care of yourself, no one else will. That's a promise.

You've read all these lessons from sexting, to BDSM, to cheating, to the grit it takes to be a single woman. They are probably overwhelming. Do you feel overwhelmed? Even I feel overwhelmed, and I'm the one who wrote it.

If you're wondering where to start, I can tell you. Just do it. You have to begin. That's where all the anxiety stems from. We psych ourselves out from doing anything and everything to avoid beginning a project. When the project is yourself, fuck, that is the most intimidating thing of all.

The best place to start in my opinion: Dump your awful boyfriend or girlfriend and send someone a sext. Sure, that's oddly specific, but I have a feeling you're somewhere on that road right now. Maybe it's a "nothing relationship" wherein the person doesn't want to put labels on it. Dump them. They suck. Perhaps it's a boyfriend or girlfriend who is always so busy and isn't a great texter. Dump them!

Another good first step: The next time someone says a shitty thing to you, don't ignore it. Now, maybe you aren't going to walk right up to a street harasser on your first go. Perhaps you won't tell your coworker that was an inappropriate comment right away. This is fine. Doing something means acknowledging it. Make a note of it in your journal and talk to a friend about it. Next time (or the next time or the next), say something.

Love yourself enough to try to make your life just a little bit better. Take back your agency because you know you deserve it. Want enough for yourself to get out there and start. As we've touched on throughout each chapter, the more rights you give a woman, the stronger she is and the more she'll act like a human being. Sexual rights are human rights. Sexual agency is something we all deserve. Start with taking back your sexuality because that is where it all starts. It is the beginning of everything. Your sexual empowerment is your resistance.

The next baby step? Masturbate. Do it regularly. Absolve yourself of sexual shame slowly, but surely. Delight in yourself. Get to know yourself. Let go of the past mistakes that haunt you. I know it's easier said than done. It always is, isn't it? Work to let them go and remind yourself, again, that you are not alone.

Next, set goals for yourself. Figure out exactly where you see yourself in the next few years. Ask for the raise you deserve. Stand up for yourself in the face of adversity. Do not ever allow anyone to make you feel badly about yourself. Ask yourself this question when you're feeling sorry for something you did or said at work: *Would I feel this way if I were a man?*

All of this is linked to your sexuality. It's the foundation for getting everything in your life in order and into a place where you feel strong, confident, and ready to take on life. You have to start somewhere. You have to start sometime. Let that sometime be today.

It is the place to begin fortifying who you are and the kind of person you want to be. If you find love, great. If you don't, don't let that bring you down. Don't see it as a failure because it isn't a failure. The only loss that counts is losing yourself to self-loathing and doubt.

We are women. We are mighty and strong and unstoppable.

We fuck who we want, when we want. No one is allowed to tell us we don't have the right to do what we want with our bodies. No one may touch you without your permission. No one may tell you anything about yourself to make you feel small.

We've got to be stronger than that. We're not alone. We are the sexually empowered, liberated women. We're in this together. The world better get the fuck ready.

Acknowledgments

I'd like to start by thanking my family. You guys are seriously the coolest and I could never be where I am if it weren't for you! Even when I wanted to write about sex and vulvas for a living, you were right there having my back all the way.

Thank you to my wonderful mom, dad, siblings, godmother, and all of my sexy fabulous friends, too! My support net has been so strong and I am eternally grateful to all of you.

Shout-out to Emily Gebhardt, Diana Reynolds, Mal Harrison, Chris Riotta, Nikolai Fedak, Teddie Austin, and Zachary Zane for always hype-gurling me so hard. You're all so crazy fabulous.

Special thanks to the Bonser family. You have all been such a force in my life and I cannot say enough to thank you. Heida, you're the bomb.

Thank you to every amazing woman (and man) in this book who shared their stories and insights with me. I'd name you all, but I know I'd miss someone and feel like a dick about it. Your voices made this book what it is and every single one of you is a BOSS.

Thank you to my amazing agents, Ashley Collom and Meg Thompson, for making this book happen in the first place. You believed in my vision and made it a reality.

Thank you to my editor and Queen of all things, Sylvan Creekmore. You edited the hell out of our baby and made it so so incredible beyond my wildest dreams.

Special thanks to Celine Rahman, for your incredible illustrations. Your clit drawings are like none other on this planet. You are a goddess.

Thank you to Julie Jones, my amazing publicist, for following me on this journey from writer to sex expert from day one. Thank you to Olivia Loving, who copyedited, like, forty proposals before we managed to sell this book to St. Martin's Press.

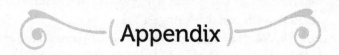

Appendix

Books

Shrill, Lindy West
I Love Female Orgasm, Dorian Solot and Marshall Miller
Cunt, Inga Muscio
The Seductive Art of Japanese Bondage, Midori
Girls & Sex, Peggy Orenstein
Come as You Are, Emily Nagoski
The Anatomy of Love, Helen Fisher
The First Sex, Helen Fisher
Mating in Captivity, Esther Perel
*Yes Means Yes! Visions of Female Sexual Power and a World Without
    Rape*, Jessica Valenti and Jaclyn Friedman
How to Be a Woman, Caitlin Moran
The Good Girls Revolt, Lynn Povich
You Are a Badass, Jen Sincero
How to Murder Your Life, Cat Marnell
The New Monogamy, Dr. Tammy Nelson
The State of Affairs, Esther Perel
Becoming Cliterate, Laurie Mintz
Shameless: A Sexual Reformation, Nadia Bolz-Weber
The Body Keeps the Score, Bessel Van der Kolk, M.D.
Men Explain Things to Me, Rebecca Solnit

Inferior: How Science Got Women Wrong and the New Research
   That's Rewriting the Story, Angela Saini
Untrue: Why Nearly Everything We Believe About Women, Lust, and
   Infidelity Is Wrong and How the New Science Can Set Us Free,
   Wednesday Martin

New Media

Why Are People Into That?!, hosted by Tina Horn
Sex 2.0 Podcast, hosted by Ian Kerner
Horizontal with Lila, hosted by Lila Donnolo
Sexology, hosted by Dr. Nazanin Maoli
Sex Out Loud, hosted by Tristan Terimino
Sex with Emily, hosted by Dr. Emily Morse
Savage Lovecast, hosted by Dan Savage
Sex with Strangers, hosted by Chris Sowa
Han and Matt Know It All, hosted by Hannah Malyn and Matt
   Albrecht